TRAUMATIC NERVE LESIONS
OF THE UPPER LIMB

Edited by J. Michon and E. Moberg

In collaboration with

E. E. Almquist, A. Bischoff, G. Bonte,
D. Brooks, O. Eeg-Olofsson, G. H. Fallet,
K. O. Fetrow, F. Iselin, H. Millesi,
G. E. Omer, J. M. Paquin, B. Petyt,
J. P. Razemon, J. Roullet, J. W. Smith,
E. Spy, R. Tubiana

First English Edition

CHURCHILL LIVINGSTONE Edinburgh London and New York 1975

CHURCHILL LIVINGSTONE

Medical Division of Longman Group Limited

Distributed in the United States of America by
Longman Inc., New York and by associated
companies, branches and representatives
throughout the world.

First edition (in French)
© Expansion Scientifique Française, 1973

First edition (in English)
© Longman Group Limited, 1975

ISBN 0 443 01057 9

Printed in Great Britain

MICHON and MOBERG

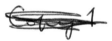

TRAUMATIC NERVE LESIONS
OF THE UPPER LIMB

Monographs of the Group d'Etude de la Main
Series edited by R. Tubiana

GROUPE D'ETUDE DE LA MAIN (G.E.M.)
List of members

Foreword

The inspiration for this monograph came from a GEM Round Table in 1969 at the Hôpital Saint-Antoine, under the chairmanship of Professor Jean Gosset, when the GEM entertained the American Society of Hand Surgery in Paris.

Among the scientific contributions to this meeting was the work of the Swedish School under Professor Erik Moberg, who has himself undertaken the task of supervising the English edition of this monograph. Our colleague Professor Verdan has supplied us with a valuable contribution resulting from a post-graduate course on nerve lesions held in Switzerland in 1970. Finally, several members of the GEM, both French and foreign, have been good enough to answer our appeal and send us the results of their experience, and this has allowed us to cover fully the subject as it stands today.

We take this opportunity to express our gratitude to all who were good enough to collaborate in this work.

The repair of the peripheral nerves remains a difficult question and we do not claim that the reports gathered here provide the final answer. In spite of all the efforts made to achieve greater technical perfection, the results when rigorously examined are still often imperfect. We hope that this volume will be a working instrument and will represent a starting point for new research and further progress.

J. Michon

Preface to the English Edition

This is the second volume to be translated into English from the series of monographs of the Groupe d'Etude de la Main. In the same way that the first volume in 1974 gave present views of authorities on Dupuytren's Disease, this volume presents a document of the current concepts of peripheral nerve injuries and their repair.

The contributions are based on papers presented in 1969 at a G.E.M. meeting in Paris and are essentially current in their approach to the classification of anatomical lesions, their investigation, prognosis and technical repair.

The recent improvements in the quality of intraneural apposition that microsurgical techniques can offer are the recurring theme of the book. Whereas pathogenesis loomed large in Dupuytren's Disease, it is intricate anatomy that dominates dissections in peripheral nerve surgery.

No excursion is attempted into the secondary reconstruction of the paralysed hand by tendon transfer or arthrodesis—these being deemed beyond the scope of the present symposium. This reconstuctive element will appear in a later volume in this G.E.M. series of monographs.

The English Edition has been prepared directly from the French and reflects the same enthusiasm for present progress and future findings that typifies the publications of the Groupe d'Etude de la Main.

1975   John Hueston

It is with very great pleasure I have accepted the suggestion of my French colleagues, especially Professor Michon, to be the co-editor for this volume. This field has through the years been one of my greatest interests. The development has rapidly advanced from a situation where it too often was believed that everything was settled. Yet today even the basic methods of examining and determining the loss and the results must be seriously questioned and scrutinized. It is no longer possible to follow the methods of neurology developed around 1890. Also, a number of totally new factors in the field of surgical technique as well as in the knowledge of the healing and maturing process has been brought into the spotlight. The activity is promising, but the goal is far ahead. Just look at the age factor. Is there any surgical field where age plays such a dominating role and so early in life?

The editors would like to thank all those who have taken such a large part in this really international work.

1975   Erik Moberg

Preface to the First Edition

The management of peripheral nerve lesions is certainly one of the most difficult and hazardous areas of reconstructive surgery. The first half of this Century was marked by lack of coordination of organized treatment, lack of precision in examination of the patient and lack of coordination in the interpretation of the results of treatment—all combining to impede progress in this important field.

The First World War emphasised the need for a systematic study of these lesions but it was only during the Second World War that definite progress was made and principally in England by the concentration of these specific injuries within centres where a concerted effort could be made towards developing methods of clinical examination and investigation, coordination of policies of management, and the development therefrom of experimental research teams. Such organization and statistical assessment of the results has been dominated now for decades by the work of Sir Herbert Seddon. It was in fact a whole decade after the war before he published the superlative summary *Peripheral Nerve Injuries* by the Nerve Injury Committee, London 1954.

Progress has continued during the past 15 years to much better effect than in that limbo between the Wars. This has been largely due to progress in specialization of surgical facilities, a wider knowledge of the specific problems of this surgery and its precise technical requirements. As a result, most of these patients are now being referred to specialized surgeons.

Moreover the generally more tidy nature of civilian nerve injuries has been better suited to the more refined facilities of civilian practice than did the wartime injuries.

For quite some time Erik Moberg and more recently Jacques Michon have been studying this field and have acquired a wide reputation in its management. They have managed to have grouped together in this monograph those authorities who have contributed to the recent advances in peripheral nerve injuries. The progress in physiology and clinical investigations is largely on the investigative and in particular the electromyographic aspects while the surgical advances are towards even greater refinements of technique and in particular the use of the operating microscope.

Finally the postoperative care of each patient has benefitted by the increased appreciation of physiological and clincial data and more efficient methods of rehabilitation.

This monograph is another collective monograph of the Group d'Etude de la Main under the supervision of two surgeons dedicated to this study, as well as the Committee on Nerve Injuries under the direction of Seddon. It has not only defined our current understanding in this field of peripheral nerve injuries but will constitute an important factor in the future development of the study and management of these injuries.

1972   Professor R. Merle d'Aubigne

Contributors

E.E.ALMQUIST Health Professional Building, Suite 701, 801 Broadway, Seattle, Washington 98122, U.S.A.

A.BISCHOFF Clinique neurologique de l'Université de Zurich, Hôpital cantonal, 8006 Zurich, Switzerland

D.BROOKS 83 Harley Street, London W1, Great Britain

G.H.FALLET Institut Universitaire de Médecine Physique et de Rééducation, Hôpital cantonal, Avenue Beauséjour, 1211 Geneva 4, Switzerland

K.O.FETROW 7905 Calumet Avenue, Munster, Indiana, U.S.A.

F.ISELIN Maison départmentale de Nanterre, Service de Chirurgie, 403 Avenue de la République, 92000 Nanterre, France.

J.MICHON Service de Chirurgie D, Hôpital Jeanne d'Arc, 54200 Dommartin-les-Touls, France

H.MILLESI Station für Plastische und Wiederherstellungchirurgie der 1 Chirurgischen, Universitäts Klinik, 1090 Vienna, Austria.

E.MOBERG Förtroligheten 50, 41270 Gothenburg, Sweden

G.E.OMER (Colonel) Chief Orthopaedic Service and Hand Surgery Center, Brooke General Hospital, Brooke Army Medical Center, Fort Sam Houston, Texas 78234, U.S.A.

J.M.PAQUIN Institut de Réadaption de Nancy, Hôpital Jeanne d'Arc, 54200 Dommartin-les-Touls, France

J.P.RAZEMON Service de Traumatologie (Pr Decoulx), Cité hospitalière, 59000 Lille, France

J.ROULLET 27 Quai Romain-Rolland, 69000 Lyon, France

J.W.SMITH 4 Sutton Place, New York, N.Y. 10022, U.S.A.

E.SPY Service de Traumatologie (Pr Decoulx), Cité hospitalière, 59000 Lille, France

R.TUBIANA 47 Quai des Grands-Augustins, 75006 Paris, France

Contents

INTRODUCTION

FUTURE HOPES FOR THE SURGICAL MANAGEMENT OF PERIPHERAL NERVE LESIONS

E. Moberg

All over the world at many well-equipped and leading centres, research work is being carried out in an attempt to improve the surgical treatment of peripheral nerve lesions. Most clinical problems involve local division of nerve branches or nerve trunks where either some kind of suture or grafting procedure obviously will be required. I will limit my remarks to those problems encountered in such cases.

It is necessary to bear in mind the very complicated macroscopic and microanatomical structure of the nerve trunk. If entirely new ways to stimulate nerve regeneration can not be found, for example, by chemical or hormonal means, then we must admit that there are obviously limits to what can be expected from merely an improvement in the surgical technique, and from a better follow-up treatment in the rehabilitation of peripheral nerve injuries. I myself am convinced that in nerve suture what can be expected from future technical improvements has already been achieved by chance in a few rare cases. In those cases we have, largely by chance, been fortunate enough to have achieved the proper alignment and tension so that follow-up has shown the optimal results. These lucky cases, however must be very rare. However, if better knowledge of the significant local neural and technical factors could help us to bring our average results up to approach the level of those few excellent results, it would mean a great step forward. Then, knowledge and the application of a reliable, good technique should be the basis for better results—rather than pure chance!

Now every discussion in this field must be based upon the exact assessment in each case of (1) the extent of motor and sensory loss and (2) the degree of recovery, the latter being calculated by the final functional result, minus the function left after loss before surgery equals the recovery obtained. Already here it must be stressed that the ninhydrin pulp printing test is of great use for determining the extent of the sensory deficit but *not* for grading the recovery. The value of forthcoming scientific papers in this field of peripheral nerve surgery will depend entirely upon the accuracy with which the assessments of loss and recovery can be measured and recorded. Any scientific paper on this subject which does not describe exactly the methods used

for determination of these two basic factors must be regarded as an unnecessary waste of scientific effort. The same applies whether a paper deals with sensory or motor recovery.

Some twenty years ago Seddon and his co-workers pointed out the clear distinction between academic recovery (examined with pinprick and cotton wool test) and functional recovery. Tachdjian and Minear, Moberg, Noordenbos, Bishop, Önne, Russell Brain, McEwan, Edshage and many others have clearly shown that the examination of sensory function by pinprick and cotton wool tests are 'rough and ready' tests which are not sufficiently accurate for comparison. They do not distinguish between tactile gnosis, paresthesia, dysethesia, hyperesthesia and similar factors and from many other points of view they are of no use for grading and evaluating sensory recovery. They are very often misleading, especially when used for determining recovery after nerve surgery. The scale Motor 1–5 may be accepted for grading motor recovery. But the scale Sensory 1–5 is useless, as real useful sensory function is only to be found between 4 and 5. It is my opinion, shared with many others, that the only test of value for this purpose is at the moment the two-point discrimination test. You may or may not agree with this view.

Today research is continuing to find better methods for testing sensory and also motor function. There is no reason why better methods should not be found when we know that those used today were developed about a century ago and for a different purpose. In this field the old sensory modality teaching must be rejected. The four modalities do not by any means cover the sensibility problems of interest to us here.

It is time therefore to insist that no paper should be accepted as a serious contribution to the problems now coming up for discussion if the author has not described in detail his method of examining and determining the original loss and the measured rate of recovery. Without such knowledge no comparison can be made with results from other workers and such papers will only give impressions, not facts.

It is also wise to remember the enormous anatomical

variations of motor and sensory fields, present in different cases especially in the hand. Again and again cases of recovery have been published, one even by myself, where obviously the loss was supposed to exist simply because a nerve was found to be cut at a certain level and according to the pictures in a textbook the function should have been lost. In fact in such cases the function often came from anomalous innervation and had never been lost, yet at the final examination has been falsely accepted as a result of nerve regeneration following the surgery.

Today a long list of factors can be made, all of potential interest, and needed for the improvement of surgical technique. Here I will outline only a few;

1. Better timing of suture or grafting.
2. Better bundle approximation at suture level:
    a. by better instruments or other technical improvements for accurate transverse cutting at time of resection
    b. by different suture technique, for example fascicular suture or intraneural bundle suture
    c. by better knowledge of bundle topography at different levels.
3. Grafting procedures; autografts, homografts, different treatment of the grafts to be inserted.
4. Vascular problems. How much can a nerve be freed without interference to its blood supply? How much can tissue fluid nutrition be relied upon? How will different grafts get revascularised?
5. Importance of surgery performed under magnification?
6. Sheathing possibilities across nerve junctions.
7. Tension problems—to find the optimum.
8. Role of immobilization and follow-up recording.
9. Improvement through specialized training.

As will be shown in another paper in this volume, the nerve conduction time as measured by electrophysiology cannot be used as a tool for determining the result. This rules out the possibility of solving many of the questions in this field by using animal experiments. Most of the work has to be done on human beings!

It has long been recognized that the age of the patient is of great importance for the result. Önne was the first one who found that, in ideal cases, a formula could be used to allow for the influence of this age factor. It must also be presumed that this age factor has the same influence in less favourable cases. Önne's ideal cases, were considered to be those in which there was very little scar tissue, where only a small nerve resection was necessary, and where no real tendon problems were present, so that a primary or early secondary suture could be performed under good local conditions provided this was by a surgeon trained in this field.

He studied the transection of the median or ulnar nerve at the wrist level, measuring recovery after five years in adults and after three years in children. He was then able to determine that the recovery given in millimetres of two-point discrimination corresponded on an average to the age in years of the patient at the time of the suture.

Therefore, to progress in this complicated and difficult field we must pick out almost ideal cases with clean cuts, little scar tissue, and correct timing of the procedure. We must divide our cases into relatively small age groups. A comparison between different cases can be made only if the level of the lesion is approximately the same. Loss and recovery must be tested by reliable methods. The precise methods used must be described in each report. We must wait at least three years in children and five years in adults to be able to claim a final result. We must test only one surgical variant at a time.

Now where in the whole world can such an enormous number of nerve lesions in suitable cases be found? I have travelled very much to find such a place. War lesions must be excluded as being too complex. My impression is that nowhere in the world is there any possibility of collecting enough cases in one single spot. Too often there are no facilities even for a fair follow-up to be made. Therefore, I believe, that our only way of getting ahead in the sensibility problems in this field will be to collect cases from several centres in the world, working on all these important problems. Then all these results according to age, level and other factors could be plotted on a curve corresponding to that of Önne, as illustrated, only when sufficient reliable material for each tested technical variation has been collected from all these different centres and correlated, may we have got a worthwhile addition to our knowledge. If the results are below the 'mean for average cases' it should mean 'no improvement on present techniques'. If the results are above this line it might mean that the technical variation has contributed an improvement. This will be the way to get precise knowledge. It will take many years but it should be possible to carry it out and it is probably the only way to advance further, namely to collect facts and not impressions. Motor recovery is less difficult but must be solved in a similar way.

Do not waste time on misdirected scientific efforts, and good luck!

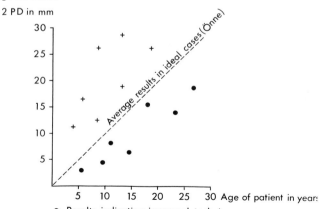

Önne's Scheme.

1. THE INTIMATE ANATOMY OF PERIPHERAL NERVES*

A. Bischoff

A peripheral nerve is composed of the neuroepithelial conducting structures and the mesenchyme which supports and protects them. For decades it was only the nerve fibre which interested anatomists and physiologists. Since they hindered experimental analysis, connective tissue and blood vessels were removed. During the Second World War, with the enormous number of wounds to limbs which had to be treated, these important structures attracted great attention in surgical operations, and fresh anatomical knowledge regarding the connective tissue sheaths of nerves and their blood circulation resulted from this. The technical development of surgery kept pace. More and more refined techniques have produced improved suture methods. Nerve homografts have been used to correct losses of tissue and the production of junctions by means of autogenous or artificial sheaths and micro-surgical techniques have all further enriched these magnificent technical developments. However, even today the results leave much to be desired. In the case of distal sutures of the ulnar nerve and the median nerve, good results are obtained in only 30 to 50 per cent of cases. What anatomical and biological conditions can be responsible for these still inadequate results?

Since the meticulous work by Cajal (1909) we have been quite familiar with the histological pattern of the nerve trunk. In cross section in most cases it appears in the form of several bundles held together by a mantle of connective tissue. Even on ordinary histological preparations under the light microscope the various parts of the nerve bundle are recognizable (Fig. 1.1). The myelinated and non-myelinated nerve fibres are surrounded by endoneural connective tissue and the perineurium, a compact sheath, isolates the endoneurium from the epineural connective tissue. Furthermore, histological sections show up some aspects of vascularization. A few large-diameter vessels are found in the epineurium and a few thin vessels—capilliaries—in the endoneurium. For the main part they are sectioned transversely, which suggests that they run along the axis of the nerve.

If we go on to study the ultrastructure of the nerve passages to which the author has devoted considerable attention (Bischoff, 1969), the high degree of resolution enables us to recognize more details of the structure of the peripheral nervous system, which has the advantage of a simple and intelligible architecture.

MYELINATED FIBRES

Each such fibre is composed of the axon surrounded by a myelin sheath, the two elements being neatly enclosed in the Schwann cell, also known as the satellite cell (Fig. 1.2).

The axon or axon cylinder is the prolongation of the nerve cell. It contains in its cytoplasm a semi-liquid gel, filaments and neurotubules, the two latter reminiscent of pipe-lines and in all probability having the same functions. At the side there are mitochondria, which are small power-plants, as well as vesicles which form part of the endoplasmic reticulum and play a role in the synthesis of cholesterol and other lipids. The axon is surrounded by its own membrane, the axolemma.

The myelin sheath, as has been known since 1950 (Fernandex-Moran), consists of lamellae arranged in a regular spiral. These are formed from the cytoplasmic membrane of the Schwann cell. The myelin sheath thus represents a membrane complex and forms part of the Schwann cell.

Knowledge of the formation of the myelin sheath is one of the great discoveries of neuro-anatomy and only became possible with the advent of the electron microscope (Geren, 1954; Robertson, 1955). In the first phase of its development the axon, still without myelin, is engulfed in the Schwann cell. This process occurs through the junction of the two cytoplasmic lips of the Schwann cell round it, forming a connection composed of the two invaginated membranes known as the mesaxon. Subsequently the mesaxon elongates and winds spirally round the axon. In the end a sleeve composed of almost 100 layers or lamellae forms the myelin sheath, which is then characterized by its periodic structure (Fig. 1.3).

Since Schwann cells are arranged in a chain, of which each link is approximately 1 millimetre long, the sheath cannot be a continuous cylinder. It is formed of segments

* The work described here was supported by the Swiss National Fund for Scientific Research (No. 4527).

3

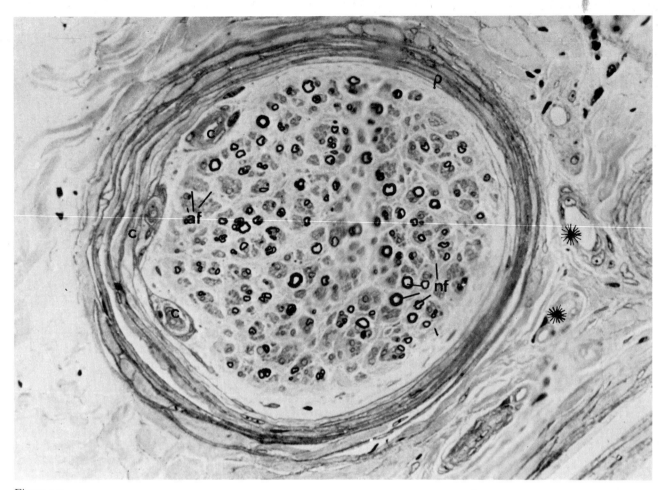

Figure 1.1
Microphotograph. Cross section of human peroneal nerve. In the endoneurium, myelinated fibres (nf) and unmyelinated fibres (af), together with capillaries (c). The perineurium (p). In the epineurium, blood vessels (⋆). Stain: methylene blue.

and each segment of the myelin sheath is as long as the Schwann cell to which it belongs. A Ranvier's node is found between each two segments, in a short unsheathed area. At this point only, the axon membrane can be stimulated through the propagation of an impulse, whereas the intermediary segment is isolated by the sheath (Robertson, 1957).

The Schwann cell, whose main function is to form the myelin sheath, is of neuro-epithelial origin. In the case of the myelinated nerve fibres there is never more than one axon surrounded by a satellite cell, whereas in the case of non-myelinated nerve fibres its relations are more complicated. In these latter fibres three different types of relationship are found:

(1) A single axon is surrounded by a satellite cell;
(2) Several axons are found in a single satellite cell;
(3) One or more axons are surrounded by two or more satellite cells, as in a sandwich.

We do not yet know the specific functions of these different types of structure. In the same way, it has so far not been possible to differentiate sensory nerve fibres from motor fibres on a morphological basis.

The Schwann cells are separated from the connective tissue by the *basement membrane*. It constitutes a barrier to diffusion without being a membrane in the proper sense of the word. This basement membrane and the nerve fibre enclosed by the Schwann cell can be distinguished from the mesenchymatous cell elements.

CONNECTIVE TISSUE

The connective tissue is conventionally (Key and Retzius, 1876) divided into three parts: the endoneurium, the perineurim and the epineurium, or, to use Louis Ranvier's terminology (1878), the intrafascicular connective tissue, the lamellar sheath and the perifascicular connective tissue.

The endoneurium comprises cells and an extracellular ground substance. Among these cells fibroblasts are the most numerous. They possess no basement membrane and are normally bigger than the Schwann cells, often forming

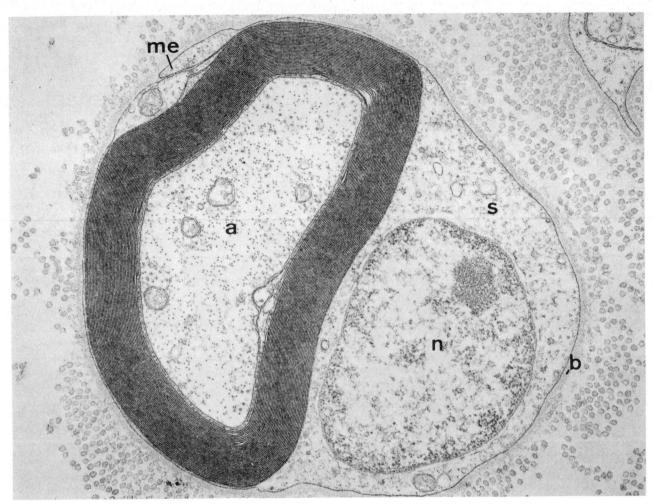

Figure 1.2
Cross-section of a myelinated fibre showing the ultrastructural pattern: the axon (a) with neurofibrils and a few mitochondria, the myelin sheath being made up by spiral arrangement of the lamellae. The two structures are ensheathed by the Schwann cell (S), here with its nucleus. The outermost lamela of the myelin sheath is connected to the Schwann cell membrane by the mesaxon (me). The Schwann cell is invested with a basement membrane (b).

very elongated cytoplasmic appendages and containing a rich array of cellular organelles. It may therefore be deduced that they possess a very high degree of metabolic activity.

Mast cells, which can be recognized by their granulation, are on the other hand not very abundant (Gamble).

The extracellular space contains collagenous fibres, which form bundles and are arranged longitudinally.

The perineurium. Each bundle is ensheathed in its own perineurium. One of the several layers of flat cells, the number corresponding to the thickness of the bundle, form the same number of extremely thin lamellae joined on the circumference. In each layer they are connected by means of compact intercellular joints and clothed in a basement membrane. Furthermore, the perineural cells are characterized by a multiplicity of micropinocytic vesicles. The principle on which they are constructed is always the same for each layer (Fig. 1.4). The structure of this perineural lamellar sheath is similar to that of a vascular endothelial wall. Moreover, this perineural tube is reinforced with collagenous fibres situated between the individual layers and orientated longitudinally, and sometimes by filaments of about 100° known as microfibrils. These are made of a sort of elastic substance and are responsible for the elasticity of the perineurium, which is orientated mainly along the axis of the nerve trunk.

The epineurium comprises all the connective tissue of the nerve trunk outside the perineurium. It is again composed of a few fibroblasts and bundles of collagenous fibres arranged for some in a circle and for some longitudinally, forming a trellis-work. Between them there are also bundles of microfibrils composed of elastic material orientated longitudinally.

A study of the connective-tissue parts of the peripheral nerve shows that they are constructed on quite different

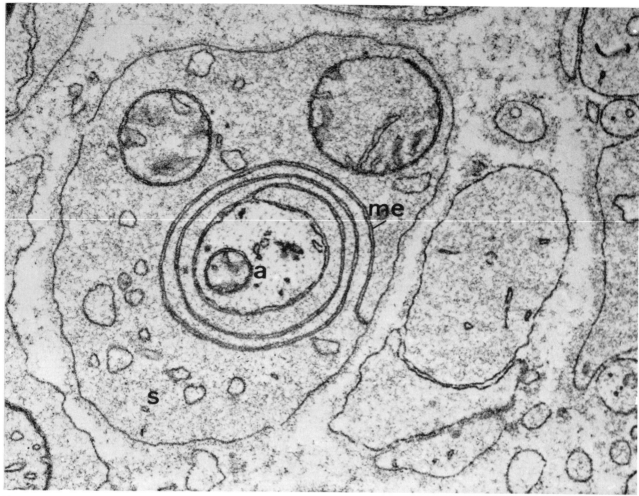

Figure 1.3
Cross-section of a nerve fibre in the peroneal nerve of a newborn mouse. It is easy to see the way in which the myelin sheath is formed by the myelin lamella (me) (formed by junction of the two membranes of the Schwann cell) being rolled round the axon (a).

principles. For this reason each of these parts has a different function.

1. The collagen bundles, situated in the endoneurium and running only longitudinally, provide the nerve fibres with protection against traction and at the same time against compression and crushing.

2. The perineural endothelial sheath has no significance from the point of view of mechanical protection. It forms a diffusion barrier (Feng and Liu; Lehmann), which from a physiological point of view might suggest that the endoneural medium probably differs from the extrafascicular medium. Indeed the endoneural medium is connected with the cerebrospinal fluid, whereas biochemically the extrafascicular resembles lymph or blood serum.

3. The main sleeve which provides mechanical protection is the epineurium, which is composed of a quite compact network of collagenous fibres. The main blood vessels of the nerve trunk are found in its mesh.

VASCULARIZATION OF THE PERIPHERAL NERVES

Electron-microscopy studies have thrown a great deal of light on the structure of the endoneural blood vessels (Bischoff). They follow a longitudinal orientation and show under the electron microscope the characteristic pattern of capillaries (Fig. 1.5), namely a ring of one or more endothelial cells resting outside on a basement membrane. Contact between them is hermetically sealed by means of intercellular junctions. A second layer of cells may be present on the outside. Against the cytoplasmic membrane of the endothelial cells are arranged the micropinocytic

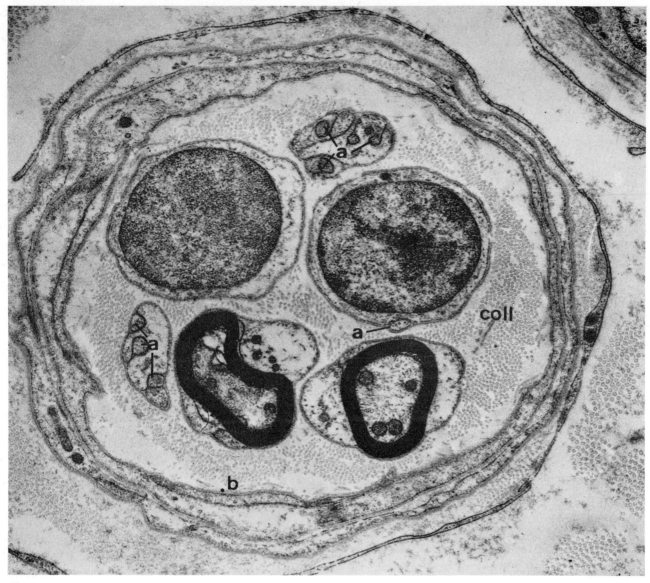

Figure 1.4
Distal segment of a peripheral nerve in cross-section, comprising two myelinated fibres and four Schwann cells with unmyelinated fibres (a). They are enclosed in the endoneural space which contains collagenous fibres (coll.). The perineurium comprises two layers of endothelial cells resting on a basement membrane (b). Outside is the epineurium, made up of a lattice of collagenous fibres.

vesicles, which are supposed to have a diffusing function. In contrast to the central nervous system there is no direct contact between the capillary and the nerve parenchyma. Between these two structures there is a free space filled with ground substance.

In addition to this feature, each nerve cord or even each branch possesses a specific and autonomous vascular network. In theory this consists of two longitudinal networks with abundant anastomoses, one extrafascicular, comprising capillaries, with collateral connections between the two networks (Fig. 1.6). The outer network is connected through *nutrient arteries* with the vascular trunks (Sunderland, 1945a). These anastomoses are usually very short, for the nerves and vascular trunks in most limb areas pursue the same course in the intermuscular spaces. They vary, however, in number and density. For example, while there are practically no anastomoses in the case of the nerves in the upper arm, several nutrient vessels arising from different main vascular trunks can be found in articular areas where the nerves are exposed to possible mechanical extension or

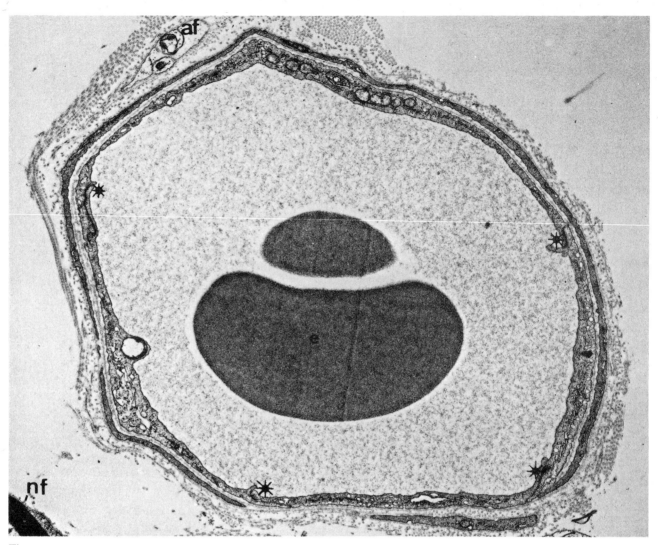

Figure 1.5
Cross section of an endoneural capillary. It is separated from the myelinated (nf) and unmyelinated (af) nerve fibres by an extracellular space. Intercellular connections (★), erythrocyte (e).

compression (Sunderland, 1945b). Thus, it is confirmed that the blood supply of nerves is by means of widely spaced external and internal anastomoses but that in very exposed areas there is an abundance of nutrient arteries to perform that task (Adams). There is convincing experimental evidence regarding the consequences of failure of a nutrient artery (Blunt, Adams). Hess, in the author's institute, has analysed and confirmed it in part. Interruption of a single nutrient artery produces neither functional disorder nor structural change. Similarly, in our experiments ligature of two nutrient arteries caused no functional disturbance. Where, for example, in the forearm the nutrient arteries are 3 to 5 centimetres apart, the nerve can be stripped over a distance of at least 6 cm. According to Roberts even the stripping of a nerve over a length of 3 cm causes no ischaemic lesion, since the intrafascicular

network is able to provide the nerve fibres with adequate nourishment. On the other hand, what *is* fatal to the blood circulation of a nerve is extension of the nerve by traction to its limit, when, as in the case of a rubber tube, its internal diameter is reduced to a very small size. In addition, blood circulation is also profoundly damaged by compression and twisting of the dissected nerve trunk.

FASCICULAR DISTRIBUTION

Modern research has made no new contribution to this problem. As a rule, the formation of nerve plexuses, as can be seen grossly in the case of the brachial plexus in the region of the shoulder girdle, extends along the whole length of the nerve to the periphery. In serial sections Sunderland (1945c) demonstrated in all nerve trunks no

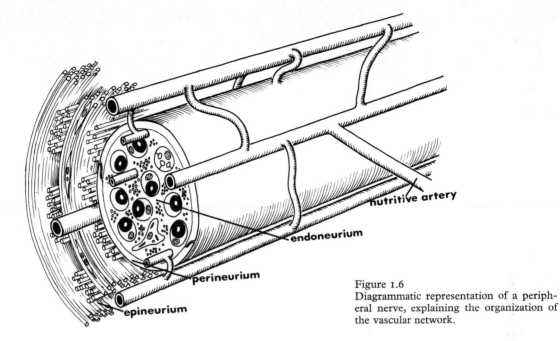

Figure 1.6
Diagrammatic representation of a peripheral nerve, explaining the organization of the vascular network.

strict relations in the order of the bundles nourished over a short distance of more than a few millimetres, or at most a centimetre. The diameter and very shape of the various bundles may change considerably. Along the whole length of a nerve, individual fibres pass from one bundle to another. Every bundle at any particular level shows a different and individual construction. The chances, therefore of finding a correspondence between the two cut surfaces of a bruised or torn nerve are slender. Furthermore, if in a mixed nerve the nerve fibres with different functions (motor, sensory, autonomic) are intermingled, it is impossible to tell from the morphological point of view to which class they belong. It is not even possible to define with certainty whether, in the various bundles, the fibres which are present are sensory or motor.

DEGENERATION AND REGENERATION OF PERIPHERAL NERVES

A divided peripheral nerve undergoes secondary degeneration throughout its distal portion, which is separated from the trophic centre. This is known as Wallerian degeneration, after the man who first observed it. It occurs as if the axon, its continuity interrupted, and the corresponding myelin sheath, were shrinking. Both are digested by the Schwann cell. Under the electron microscope the process becomes visible about 24 hours after sectioning and reaches its peak after about 7 days. It can, however, last several weeks before it comes to an end. Whereas the axon and myelin sheath are destroyed and disappear, the

Schwann cell survives. It remains in a belt of cells known as Büngner's band.

Regeneration of the nerve fibre is shown by sprouting of the central portion, which can be seen as early as 3–4 days after sectioning. If these buds encounter cords of Schwann cells they will be invaginated by them and remyelinated, depending on their origin. The remyelination process follows the same rules as myelination in ontogenesis. Schwann cells preserve their capacity for remyelination for years (Sunderland, 1952). The axons which do not come into contact with the remaining Schwann cells will undergo atrophy and retraction later. This occurs particularly when they become lost in the extrafascicular connective tissue.

Whether axon budding succeeds or not depends above all on the axons encountering Schwann cells, i.e. whether they find their original path in the endoneurium. The higher the number of Büngner bands available, the greater the probability of regeneration. Similarly in the case of autografts, the larger the endoneural canal, the greater the chances that the rebudding axons will encounter Büngner bands and not become lost in the interfascicular connective tissue (Smith, 1900: Sunderland, 1954; Sunderland and Ray).

Two obstacles may hinder this regeneration, viz.:
(1) The use of too small a bundle for grafting, with too few Büngner's bands; (2) Barriers in the way of regeneration consisting of debris or proliferating connective tissue.

Considering the small number of endoneural fibroblasts, it is obvious that in cases of nerve-trunk damage the fibroblasts of the epineural sheath enter the endoneurium. They are stimulated by the change in the chemical milieu inside the bundle, which now contains blood serum as the result of the rupture of blood vessels.

The conclusions drawn in regard to therapy should be as follows: (1) Every bundle should be individually sutured, and it should be sutured to a graft bundle of large enough diameter; (2) The bundles should be sutured hermetically in view of the fact that the perineurium is an endothelial tissue constituting a diffusion barrier. The reason for this is that this lamellar sheath affords protection against the lower osmotic difference inside the membrane. Artificial fixation of the suture on the outside is therefore pointless and if it is carried out with a permeable membrane, even harmful; (3) The suture must not be under tension. Any tension on the suture may reopen the closed perineural sheath and hinder the circulation, by traction on the vessels lying longitudinally.

2. VARIATIONS IN SENSORY NERVE SUPPLY TO THE HAND

Kenneth O. Fetrow

The purpose of this paper is to call attention to the fact that individual variations in the fields covered by different nerves in the hand are present to an extent much greater than that which is usually described in the literature. These variations are of great practical significance in surgery of the hand.

The hand is a most important sensory organ and its skin, particularly on the palmar surface, is abundantly supplied with all types of sensory receptors. A detailed knowledge of the variation of distribution of sensory cutaneous nerves of the hand and digits is of considerable clinical importance. It is chiefly by knowledge of the fields of sensory manifestations that treatment and prognosis of a lesion can be handled appropriately. It must be stressed that for surgery of the hand it is of little importance to distinguish between the so-called autonomous and the maximal field of innervation from a certain nerve. Neither are the old-time terms 'protopathic' and 'epicritic' sensibility linked in such a way with those factors important for hand surgery that it is worthwhile to use them. It is now known that the areas of tactile gnosis, the ability to identify objects by touch alone without visual perception, are almost identical to the areas with a normal two-point discrimination. Tactile gnosis and two-point discrimination are the factors which are of practical value for use in hand surgery. When a nerve is divided, there is a borderline between the area which has lost tactile gnosis and the surrounding parts where the tactile gnosis is intact. This borderline stays where it is and will not change even during decades, if surgical means are not undertaken in order to change the situation (Moberg).

Early after nerve transection there is a shrinking of that area supplied solely by the transected nerve and extension of that area overlapped by the transected nerve and the nerves adjacent to it, from ingrowth of nerve fibres from nearby uninvolved normal nerves (Foerster). This type of sensibility does not give tactile gnosis. Sensibility resulting from ingrowth of neighbouring nerves should be clearly distinguished from 'true' sensory regeneration with a return of tactile gnosis. Where there is doubt, the adjacent nerves may be blocked and, if the sensibility is due to ingrowth, it will disappear, but if it is due to regeneration, it will be unaffected (Önne).

Considerable useful information with regard to the variation in distribution of cutaneous nerves is omitted from the standard textbooks of anatomy. The reason for this, of course, is because it is not possible to determine the exact distribution of sensory nerve supply to the hand by the crude method of anatomical dissection. The few facts available are not linked with tactile gnosis and, therefore, are of limited value for surgery. Most textbooks describe the different fields of innervation in the ways shown in the following figures of the dorsal and volar aspect of the hand (Fig. 2.1).

The median nerve sensation to the thumb is supplied by: (a) The proper lateral digital nerve of the thumb which supplies the pulp of the radial side of the thumb and the dorsal subungual area; and (b) The proper medial digital nerve of the thumb supplying the ulnar side of the thumb pulp and the subungual region of the tip. The radial nerve sensation to the thumb is supplied by the superficial radial nerve, lateral and medial branches, which supplies the dorsum of the thumb, radial and ulnar aspect respectively, but not the subungual area (Gray). Normally the boundary follows the midlateral line, but occasionally quite a large part of the pulp may be supplied by the superficial radial nerve (Moberg).

The volar surface of the ring finger is ordinarily innervated by the median and ulnar nerves. The boundary between the area supplied by these two nerves usually follows the midline of the palmar aspect of the ring finger although variability is present here also. Either the median or ulnar nerve may supply the whole of the cutaneous palmar surface of this finger. Stopford, in a large series of cases, stated that the ulnar nerve supplied the whole of the palmar surface of both the ring and little fingers in about 18 per cent of his cases while the median nerve supply of the total palmar surface of the ring finger was 4 per cent of his series of patients. Stopford tested only 'epicritic sensibility' with the use of a fine camel hair brush. Wynn Parry states that 5 per cent of patients with peripheral nerve injuries had either median or ulnar nerves supplying the whole of the ring finger. However, he does not give his clinical method of determination. McEwan has reported as an incidental finding an extreme example of thumb pulp

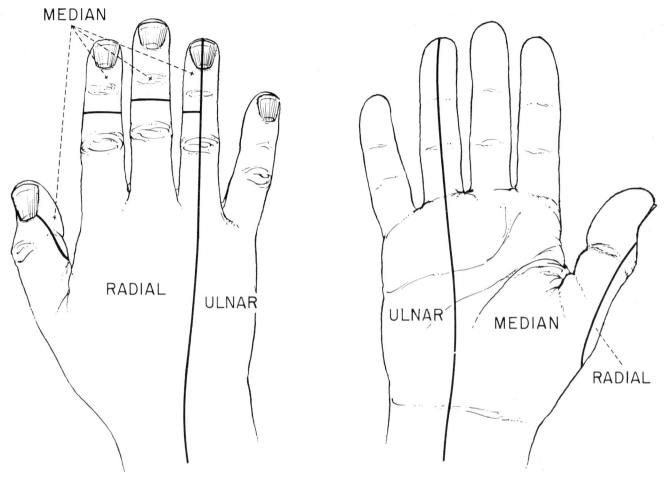

Figure 2.1 Fields of innervation of the hand:

A, Dorsal aspect   B, Palmar aspect.

almost totally innervated by the radial digital dorsal branches while investigating median and ulnar nerve injuries using the ninhydrin test (McEwan). Other examples of the great variations and their value in reconstructive surgery are given by Moberg. However, no systematic survey has been performed so far on the great variations of sensory innervation of the thumb.

It is of the utmost importance to be aware of the variations of the nerve supply of the hand and to understand the sometimes complex nature of the variations in injuries of the hand in order to plan and carry out the proper surgical treatment. It is also important to evaluate properly an injured hand pre-operatively so that following the surgical procedure the return of function and/or sensation may be assessed using the pre-operative status as the baseline. On occasion, the injured hand may possess certain findings pre-operatively that were not properly evaluated and, hence, attributed to the surgical procedure in the post-operative assessment.

It is, therefore, of interest to study the variations of tactile gnosis or sensory innervations of the pulp of the thumb because of the great individual variations of innervation from the radial nerve (Moberg).

Ordinarily, the radial nerve will supply the skin on the dorsum of the thumb as well as on the sides of the thumb nail with some branches overlapping onto the volar aspect of the thumb in varying degrees. Therefore, total loss of median nerve sensory function when limited to the thumb will be noticed little if the radial nerve overlap onto the thumb pulp is sufficient. In a median nerve lesion at wrist level, such a thumb will also retain an almost normal function against the ring finger and little finger if the thenar muscles are supplied by the ulnar nerve enough to give fair opposition (Moberg). (Fig. 2.2).

If, however, there is no sensory supply or only a minimal sensory supply from the radial nerve to the thumb pulp, the thumb grip will be unsatisfactory even with functional grip muscle power. In median nerve lesions with complete

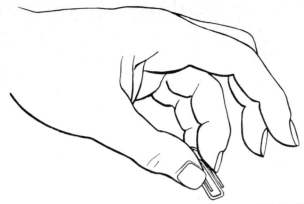

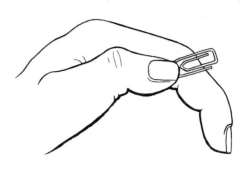

Figure 2.2
The precision sensory grip present in median nerve sensory loss where thumb pulp is adequately supplied by radial nerve overlap, and where sufficient motor function for opposition is present.

Figure 2.3
Thumb grip against dorsolateral border of proximal phalanx of index (radial nerve) in a patient lacking radial nerve innervation to the thumb pulp and lacking opposition (median nerve loss).

(Figures 2.2 and 2.3 reproduced by courtesy of Professor Moberg and the Editor of the *Bulletin of the Hospital for Joint Diseases*.)

loss of opposition, the motor function of the thumb will depend on the adductor pollicis, the extensor pollicis longus (also very useful as an adductor) and the flexor pollicis longus. In this instance, without radial nerve overlap to the thumb pulp, grasping will take place between the side of the distal phalanx of the thumb and the dorsoradial side of the base of the index finger innervated by the radial nerve, but this grip is poor for small objects. The hand will, therefore, often use the ring finger against the little finger for its best precision grip (Fig. 2.3).

MATERIAL AND METHODS

This investigation was carried out by clinical methods and nerve block experiments rather than psychophysical methods.

Thirty volunteer adult patients were used in this study. No children were used. Some patients with complete median nerve lesions were used. No nerve suture cases were used. In this paper only normal variations are discussed. The ninhydrin printing test was used in this work to demonstrate the areas of sensation supplied by the radial, median, and ulnar nerves. The ninhydrin test is the best test to determine the definite borders of the sensory areas of the hand as no co-operation by the patient is needed. However, technical accuracy is necessary. Pins and cotton wool were not used as they do not differentiate between paraesthesiae and sensibility. Two point discrimination was not used as it is difficult to perform this test on the narrow border zones of the thumb and ring finger and the patient must be fully co-operative.

If there was no lesion of the median nerve, regional median nerve block was done at the wrist level using 2 per cent carbocaine with adrenalin. After satisfactory anaesthesia was obtained, ninhydrin prints were carefully taken.

The radial nerve was then blocked at the wrist level with 2 per cent carbocaine with adrenalin and prints taken and, in some cases, the ulnar nerve was blocked at the sulcus nervi ulnaris also using 2 per cent carbocaine with adrenalin and prints again taken. A set of initial prints was taken prior to any nerve block.

If a total median nerve lesion was present, the median nerve block was obviously omitted, but initial prints were taken and then the radial and/or ulnar nerve block was performed and repeat prints taken to determine the amount of sensation, if any, present in the sensory distribution of the nerve.

Sweat glands are supplied by sympathetic fibres entering the anterior primary rami of the brachial plexus and following the sensory pathways to the periphery. Division or interruption of a sensory nerve by trauma or with local anaesthesia nerve block results in anhidrosis in its field of distribution. The extent of the anhidrosis is easily demarcated by feeling with the finger as the surface is dry and smooth. This gives a simple method of clinical examination. However, for a more objective examination, the ninhydrin test is especially suitable for clinical use (Moberg). The ninhydrin prints were obtained by pressing the pulp of the fingers, one at a time, slowly and steadily against a strip of clean, untouched paper that does not contain materials stainable with ninhydrin, measuring 3 by 15 centimetres. The fingertip outline was traced on the paper with a lead pencil that contained no soluble dye. In the case of fingers with double sensory innervation, as the thumb and ring finger, it was useful to roll the finger from one side of the nail margin to the other to get both the radial and ulnar borders (Fig. 2.4).

The fingerprints are then developed by either one of two methods. The fingerprints may be developed by spraying the paper with a 0·2 per cent solution of ninhydrin and acetone aerosol spray followed by heating the paper in an

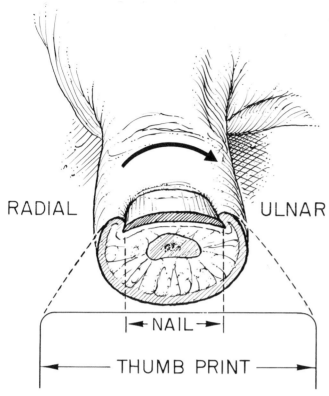

Figure 2.4
The thumbprint is obtained by rolling the finger from one nail margin to the other, in order to secure a print having both a radial and an ulnar border.

oven at 100°C for 3 to 5 minutes. The second method is to dip the paper in a 1 per cent ninhydrin acetone solution acidified with a few drops of glacial acetic acid per 10 millilitres. This solution is stable for only about a week. The prints are then developed by drying at 100° to 120°C for 5 minutes. The ninhydrin reacts with the amino acid and the lower peptides present in the sweat to produce purple dots. These dots merge to form patches when the secretion is increased or if the technique is faulty. During the next twenty-four hours there is some intensification. After this period of time the prints may be fixed in a 1 per cent copper nitrate solution acidified with a few drops of concentrated nitric acid per 100 millilitres and these prints will remain stable for a period of several years. In addition, for permanent fixation, a photographic record (xerox) of the developed fingerprints can be carried out and the prints will be stable and unchangeable. In patients over 45 years of age, the sweat secretion is often not intense enough to give readable prints and it may be necessary to stimulate their sweat secretion by giving them a cup of tea or having them exercise for 5 minutes. It also may be necessary to wipe the fingers clean with ether prior to taking the prints in order to get a good set of readable prints. Moberg (1958), pointed out that the fingerprint test is unlikely to be of

value in very high brachial plexus lesions or when there has been injury to or operation on the sympathetic chain. All acute injuries and infections have an inhibitory effect on sudomotor activities though there is not total anhydrosis such as is found after complete division of the nerve (Önne). No such complications were present in the cases presently examined.

RESULTS

Ordinarily, it is thought that radial nerve sensation is confined to the dorsum of the thumb and above the midlateral line, but not including the subungual area. However, the radial nerve innervation past the midlateral line onto the volar pulp may be sufficient so that following total median nerve lesion there is adequate sensation of the thumb to allow a good pinch function. In a large proportion of cases, it is seen that the pulp of the thumb has a good volar innervation from the radial nerve overlap from the dorsum of the thumb. Therefore, in spite of median nerve sensory loss following injury, the thumb may be quite useful. Thirty patients were evaluated using the ninhydrin test to determine the radial nerve innervation (tactile gnosis) onto the volar surface of the thumb. There is no absolutely accurate way to give in figures the size of the areas with and without tactile gnosis. However, the ninhydrin fingerprinting test will define the area of tactile gnosis and can be used to determine loss and presence of tactile gnosis, giving the borderlines between the different areas involved very accurately. The volar field of radial nerve innervation present after loss of median function has been measured in millimetres from the radial and ulnar margins of the thumb nail. The numerical values are given in Fig. 2.5 and show the distribution of the variations. In

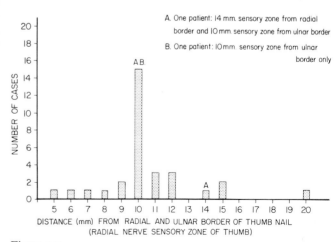

Figure 2.5
Cutaneous radial nerve variation of the thumb A, One patient: 14 mm sensory zone from radial border and 10 mm sensory zone from ulnar border B, One patient: 10 mm sensory zone from ulnar border only.

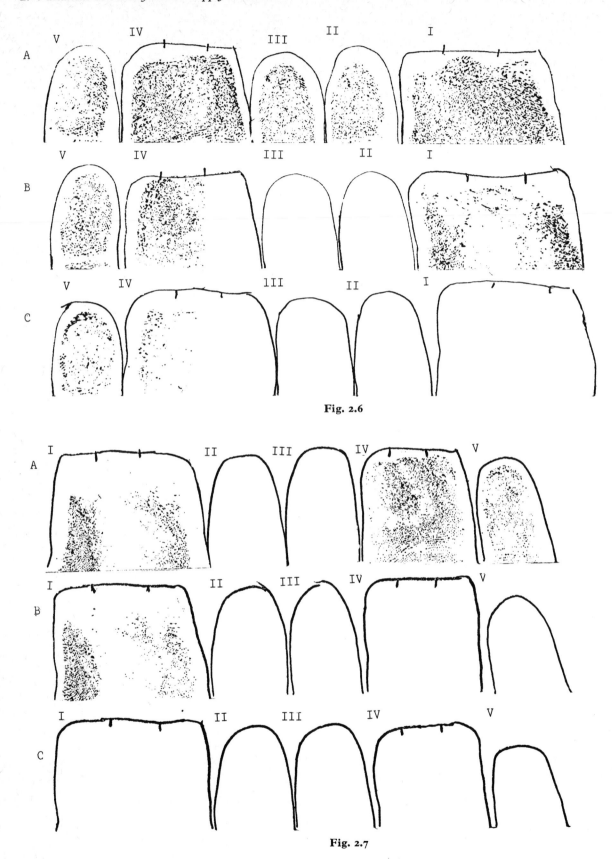

Fig. 2.6

Fig. 2.7

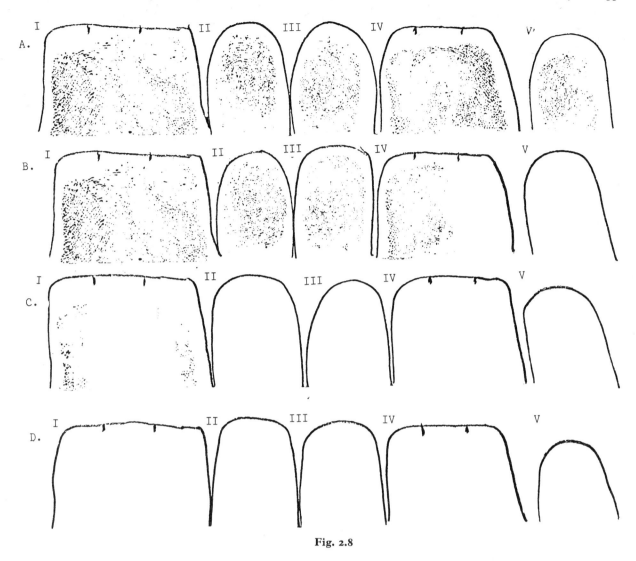

Fig. 2.8

Figure 2.6
Patient A.A. A, Pre-block; shows normal sensation; B, After median nerve block; sensory loss primarily index, middle and partially ring finger. Extensive radial nerve sensation of thumb; C, After median and radial nerve block; sensation remains only partial ring and 5th finger (ulnar nerve sensation).

Figure 2.7
Patient R.P. Traumatic median nerve resection at wrist; A, Pre-block; radial nerve sensation present on thumb. Ulnar nerve supplied entire ring finger; B, Ulnar nerve block; only radial nerve sensation present on thumb; C, Radial and ulnar nerve block; digits anaesthetic.

Figure 2.8
Patient R.S. A, Pre-block; normal sensation; B, Ulnar nerve block; C, Ulnar and median nerve block; minimal radial nerve innervation to thumb; D, Radial, median, ulnar nerve block; digits anaesthetic.

this series of patients, the variability ranged from 5 millimetres to 20 millimetres radial nerve sensation, being measured from both the radial and ulnar borders of the nail margin, with one-half of the patients having a 10 millimetre sensory zone from the radial and ulnar border of the thumb and onto the volar surface of the thumb. Two patients with median nerve injuries had a 15 millimetre and 12 millimetre sensory zone respectively, on either side of the thumb nail and could function well in grasping objects even though they had absent median nerve sensation to the thumb.

The prints of AA, KS and RP (Figs. 2.6, 2.7, 2.8) show the maximal and minimal fields covered by the radial, median and ulnar nerves in the thirty random cases: RP had a complete transection of the median nerve at wrist level.

Five of the thirty patients had the cutaneous sensation to the ring finger supplied totally by the median nerve while two patients of the thirty patients had cutaneous sensibility of the ring finger supplied totally by the ulnar nerve.

SUMMARY

When injury occurs to nerves of the hand, division into areas of complete and partial loss of sensibility is of less interest than detailed knowledge of the normal anatomical ranges of variation. For several years it has been clinical observation that when a nerve is severed, the sensory disturbance affects a cutaneous area varying considerably between different people. Great individual variations in innervation from the radial nerve to thumb pulp are common. In the thumb, the border zones of the radial nerve are of the utmost importance, especially after median nerve injury and when planning reconstructive surgery. The border zones of the radial nerve are often different on the radial and ulnar sides of the thumb. The ulnar side, of course, is the most important side.

Thirty patients were examined using the ninhydrin test for radial nerve overlap onto the volar aspect of the thumb into the area of what is usually thought of as median nerve sensation. There was considerable variability present in the patients examined with the radial nerve innervation on both the radial and ulnar border of the thumb nail averaging 10 millimetres in the majority of patients. This amount of 'overlap' is an important consideration when planning reconstructive procedures on the thumb and for assessing satisfactory function of the hand.

ACKNOWLEDGEMENT

It is with gratitude that I acknowledge the privilege of being able to spend several months with Professor Erik Moberg and to have had the opportunity to carry out this work under his supervision. Also, I would like to acknowledge the International College of Surgeons who helped make this postgraduate study possible.

Figs. 8 and 9 are reproduced with the permission of Professor Eric Moberg and the Editor of the *Bulletin of the Hospital for Joint Diseases*.

3. ELECTROMYOGRAPHY IN PERIPHERAL NERVE INJURIES

J. M. Paquin

Rehabilitation requires a precise knowledge of the condition of the muscles. Clinical examinations and tests have certain limits and biopsy is not a simple technique. An over-all electromyogram with skin surface electrodes, ordinary electromyography, study of action potentials after stimulation, and calculation of conduction velocities, provides information which makes it possible to refine the diagnosis.

In rehabilitation work we take this into account, in order to prescribe a course of treatment which extends from reception at the Centre until occupational activities are fully resumed.

Among the applications of the EMG, we shall mention its contribution to the diagnosis and prognosis in lesions of the peripheral nerves and in muscular atrophy. We shall say a little on electromyography in the study of surgical stumps, but nothing of its part in motor disorders originating in the central nervous system or essential scoliosis. We must point out, however, that examinations carried out so far in the latter have provided no useful information.

Of the last 600 EMGs that we have carried out, half were requested for the purpose of more precise diagnosis and for prognosis in lesions of the lateral popliteal, radial, median and ulnar nerve trunks. Roughly one quarter were carried out to determine the cause of lesions of obscure origin. There were twenty cases of brachial plexus traction injury of traumatic or obstetrical origin, and the same number before or after muscle transfers. Four patients had a leg amputation, a few cases had Guillain-Barré syndrome or myopathies, and a few cases had Volkmann's paralysis.

Lesions of major nerve trunks may be open or closed. Following open injuries by sharp objects, the nerve may be partially or completely sectioned. In the case of total section followed by secondary surgical suture, clinical signs will give us information on the recovery of sensory function (Tinel's sign, sensitivity test, ninhydrin test). Electromyograms following stimulation will enable detection of the first signs of re-innervation at a moment when clinical tests are still negative. Subsequently, electromyography will make it possible to follow the development of the re-innervation.

An electromyogram with numerous small potentials provides a favourable prognosis, whereas repeated readings with few potentials at high frequency indicate a rather unfavourable prognosis, particularly if it is found that the potentials progressively increase in amplitude.

Following an open injury, the nerve is sometimes only partially sectioned. In such cases thorough examination will provide information on the extent and topography of the lesion and make it possible to decide whether to operate or not.

Following a closed injury, the case history will supply information on whether there is heavy and transient bruising (a blow, tourniquet, etc.) or whether there has been slow compression (callus or scar). When the history of the accident suggests injury to the nerve from contusion, the conduction velocity makes it possible to assess the general or partial nature of the nerve lesion, provided, of course, that the nerve can still be excited, and by comparison with the healthy side, supernormal stimulation will provide us with information regarding the extent of the lesion.

I shall recall here Seddon's physiological classification of nerve injuries.

Neuropraxia: loss of axon conduction but no lesion of the nerve sheath and no rupture of the axon.

Axonotmesis: degeneration of the endoneural sheath with marked axonic discontinuity with loss of conduction until the axon has regenerated.

Neurotmesis: physiological sectioning of the total nerve sheath and trunk with loss of conduction which makes surgical reconstruction essential.

In certain cases with progressive atrophy of some groups of muscles, the X-ray and clinical examination may suggest a compression of the nerve by a callus or scar. Serial electromyograms sometimes reveal a gradual reduction in the number of motor units, indicating the need for surgical operation.

The EMG will therefore provide the rehabilitation team with information on the extent of the lesion, the appearance of the first signs of re-innervation and the outcome of the paralysis.

We have often been asked for electromyograms in cases with a picture of atrophy and functional disability.

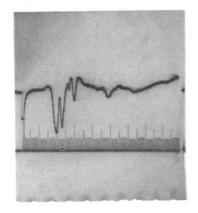

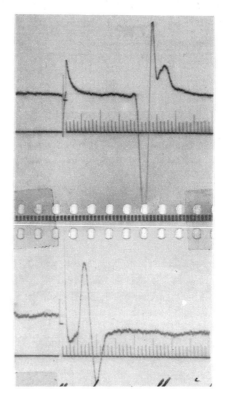

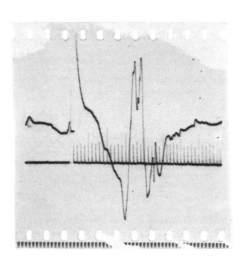

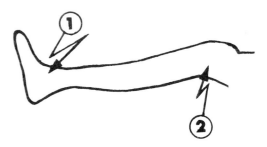

Figure 3.1
Techniques of stimulation and detection. (a) *May 1970*: low fracture of the femur complicated by paralysis of the peroneal nerve. *September 1970*: stimulation of the peroneal nerve in the popliteal fossa. Polyphasic response of the re-innervation type in the upper part of the tibialis anterior. (b) *15 August 1970*: injury to the front of the knee. Steppage gait at the end of the day. *October 1970*: stimulation of the peroneal nerve. Polyphasic response of the neuritis type in the extensor digitorum brevis.

Figure 3.2
Lead electrodes. Measurement of the conduction velocity of the motor fibres of the lateral popliteal nerve. The response was obtained in the extensor digitorum brevis muscle.
1. Stimulation of the lower point.
2. Stimulation of the upper point.

In some patients with muscular atrophy found by the rehabilitation team, electromylgraphic examination will disclose whether this is simply atrophy through disuse, reflex atrophy in response to pain, neurogenic atrophy or primary myogenic atrophy. A long period of inaction brings in its train only minor electromyographic changes, such as a high number of short motor units or polyphasic motor units, but the EMG gives a reading which is well correlated with the effort exerted. Sometimes in such cases it will be well correlated with the effort exerted. Sometimes in such cases it will be advantageous to make the muscle work through using its fixative or stabilizing functions. In the case of pain syndromes, the patient will not contract his muscles to any extent because he is afraid of the pain, but the reading obtained correlates with the contraction. Often a tendency towards a grouping of the motor units will be observed. Such readings are easily differentiated from the readings resulting from neurogenic atrophy and those caused by myogenic atrophy.

Sometimes I am asked to examine persons with a muscular deficiency which they ascribe to an old injury. The electromyogram may show up neurogenic atrophy marked by large action potentials with a high frequency. When considerable deformity is present the EMG will show the contribution made by contracture (shown objectively by activity at rest) and the part attributable to fibromusculotendinous retractions.

In Volkman's syndrome the EMG is of practical value for determining the contribution made by any contracture that may be present compared with that by musculotendinous retraction and that ascribable to median nerve injury. When the pattern is dominated by retraction and contracture, a test reading will be obtained which is notably improved if traction is exerted on the fingers. On the other hand, when nerve injury is the dominant element, examination of the small muscles of the hand and the muscles of the forearm will make it possible to obtain a complete picture of the areas served by the median, ulnar and radial nerves.

It should be noted that in examination of a patient with scapulohumeral periarthritis the EMG will show the presence of 'silent zones' in some muscles, as well as zones with numerous brief potentials of low amplitude.

Out of 600 persons examined, we had 20 branchial lesions of the brachial plexus. In root lesions the EMG findings indicate the radicular topography of the damaged motor nerves and demonstrate fibrillation, which is one of the best localizing signs. Often the damage is very severe and re-innervation is very late and functional recovery poor. Repeated EMGs enable us to follow what is happening and suggest when palliative surgical operations or muscle transplants may be helpful.

Sometimes two or three years after the accident an EMG will enable us to sum up the situation and may suggest that amputation is to be considered.

In birth palsy the EMG often makes it possible to determine the extent of the paralysis and to follow its evolution. At the sequelae stage it demonstrates in muscles which are clinically supernormal traces of chronic neurogenic atrophy with potentials of large amplitude.

In traumatic paralysis and birth palsy, the EMG will demonstrate objectively the reciprocal innervation which partly explains the disability finally observed.

I have also carried out a certain number of electromyographic examinations to estimate the value of possible tendon transfers. The EMG shows whether the muscle has undergone partial denervation and can be recovered without any apparent clinical signs. Indeed, if a muscle which is partly denervated is chosen for a transplant, it may happen that its removal will involve further denervation, or that the effort demanded after transplantation overloads the damaged muscle.

After tendon transfers, electromyography makes it possible to observe the behaviour of the transferred muscle. In the case of radial nerve paralysis we have been able to follow the development of different transfers, such as the pronator teres, the flexor carpi ulnaris muscle, or the palmaris longus. I have a small device which enables the patient to see for himself the contraction of the transplanted muscle.

The EMGs which I have done on leg stumps were designed to measure the activity of the sectioned muscles and to compare what happens in a stump after osteomyoplasty. The results obtained were very disappointing, since in four cases of amputation I found a reading showing neurogenic atrophy in the muscles of the anterolateral compartment of the leg.

In conclusion, the EMG supplies information of several kinds.

It provides data on the extent of the nerve injury and makes it possible to detect the first signs of re-innervation.

It shows the effect of the treatment, not only surgical but particularly of re-education.

In particular, successive examinations may reveal the persistence of a featureless EMG so that the prognosis is unfavourable, or they may show a more varied pattern with a favourable prognosis. Information is thus obtained on the direction in which the atrophy is developing.

The EMG detects the first signs of re-innervation in the phase of regeneration of nerve trunk lesions or after nerve suture, when a needle inserted in a clinically inactive muscle can record incipient re-innervation potentials

The EMG enables us to assess the value of methods of rehabilitation, particularly in the case of tendon transfers.

After damage to the nerve trunks then, a featureless electromyogram shows that nerve conduction persists.

The absence of signs of re-innervation after a certain period has elapsed justifies surgical intervention.

In the case of nerve sutures, the EMG will detect the first signs of re-innervation and make it possible to follow its development. If, after a certain period, a featureless reading is obtained with hypertrophied motor unit, it is easy to deduce that only a few axons have become reconnected to the muscle and the functional prognosis is poor, while the opposite is the case if after a certain time a trace rich in motor units is recorded, from which it may be deduced that recovery will be good.

In the case of nerve compression by a callus or scar, the EMG makes it possible to follow its progressive development, which may justify the freeing of the nerve.

Combination of electromyography with nerve stimulation makes it possible to differentiate organic lesions from hysterical or simulated lesions.

In combination with technical procedures it contributes to the rehabilitation of the disabled and provides a better understanding of the part played by the different muscle groups.

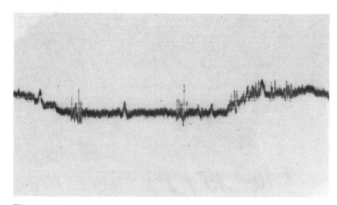

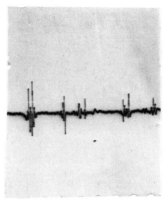

Figure 3.3
Suture of the lateral popliteal nerve at the beginning of July 1970.
   Electromyogram recorded at the beginning of October 1970.
It shows very small polyphasic re-innervation potentials.

Figure 3.4
Radial nerve paralysis after fracture of the humerus. The EMG
was taken at the end of September, 6 months after the accident.

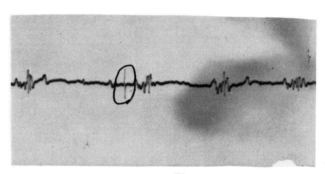

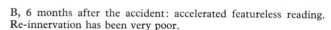

Figure 3.5
Small re-innervation potentials.
Dislocation of the shoulder, circumflex paralysis.

A, 4 months after the accident, small re-innervation potentials.
A denervation potential is also recorded with a 0.

B, 6 months after the accident: accelerated featureless reading.
Re-innervation has been very poor.

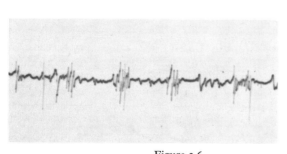

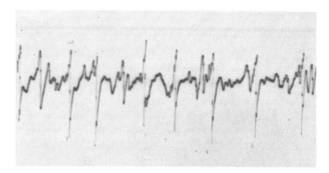

Figure 3.6
Successive traces obtained after suture of the median nerve in the
wrist.

B, 6-7 months after rehabilitation: trace of the intermediate type.
A potential will be noted with a frequency a little above 20 per
second.

A, 4 months afterwards: quite numerous polyphasic potentials in
the opponens muscle.

The final result was quite good. The remaining motor units were
hypertrophied.

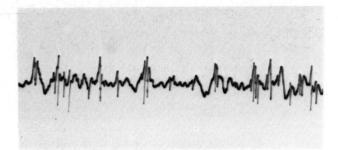
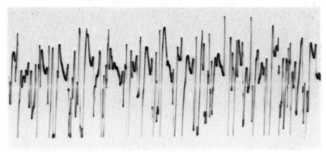

Figure 3.7
Successive recordings in the extensor carpi radialis longus after
radial nerve paralysis through compression during sleep.

A, 3 weeks afterwards: numerous potentials.

B, 2 months afterwards: recording rich in motor units.
Functional recovery was complete.

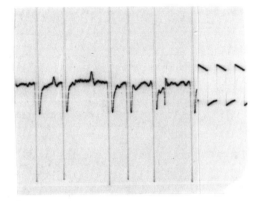
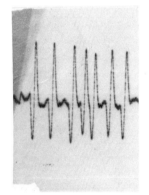

Figure 3.8
Accelerated featureless trace
Mrs K., EMG taken in October 1970 with a unipolar lead in the
hypothenars.
Rate of movement of the camera: 250 mm/sec.
Reference: 100

Figure 3.9
Very much accelerated featureless trace
The EMG was taken in the biceps 18 months after stretching of
the brachial plexus due to injury.

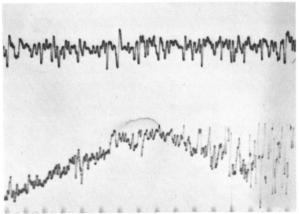

Figure 3.10
Ten-year-old child—birth palsy. The upper line corresponds to
the biceps, the lower line to the triceps.
The recording was obtained during an attempt at flexing the arm.
The contraction of the triceps hinders the working of the biceps.
This defect in re-innervation makes functional recovery doubtful.

4. THE PROGNOSTIC VALUE OF CLINICAL ELECTROMYOGRAPHY

E. Spy and J. P. Razemon

The value of an EMG study of a nerve trunk lesion depends on the investigator's experience of this technique and his knowledge of its potentialities.

These become more extensive from day to day but demand close co-operation between surgeons and electromyologists. The electromyologist is not only unaware of most surgical techniques, which is excusable, but also of the surgeon's intentions, and reports either vaguely to the questions he is asked or even irrelevantly, thus throwing undeserved discredit on a method that is of great value provided that its indications and limits are recognized.

It is now 15 years since the EMG began to be applied in clinical practice. Its applications are particularly important in investigating peripheral nerve lesions, as has been emphasized by Bauwens in Britain, Buchthal in Denmark, Dumoulin in Belgium, Marinacci and Licht in the U.S.A., and Lerique and Isch in France.

The value of the EMG lies in the diagnostic and prognostic information it provides. We shall deliberately leave aside the technical aspects, physiological considerations and anomalies of re-innervation and deal only with its practical indications.

DIAGNOSTIC VALUE

In the case of an open wound an electromyographic examination is unnecessary, since the pattern of nerve lesions can be determined at the same time as the wound is explored and repaired.

In the case of a closed wound, or one already repaired, the EMG provides several additional aspects of information.

In the early stage, before Wallerian degeneration has taken place (21 days) and while electrical examination by stimulation still produces normal results, it will show the extent and distribution of the neurogenous deficiency.

The loss of motor units is shown: during effort, by reduction in the number of motor unit potentials and an increase in their frequency to compensate for the dropping-out of the paralyzed units; at rest, by spontaneous fibrillation.

Each of these two phenomena differs in degree according to the extent of the deficiency, thus providing a means of estimating it quantitatively.

In attempts to determine the extent of the deficiency the EMG proves useful when clinical diagnosis is difficult, i.e. when the pattern is atypical either in the case of partial section or in that of recent injury with oedema and stiffness, which make mobilization difficult and prevent the performance of muscle tests.

This quantitative investigation provides a picture of the *topography* of the deficiency and pinpoints the site of the lesion.

In a person with multiple injuries, for example, ulnar paralysis when found may be due either to the wound which is at the moment closed and can be seen in the forearm, or to a nerve trunk lesion at a higher level. An electromyographic investigation in detail provides an answer by revealing in the case of higher lesions, neurogenic changes, often clinically concealed, above the wound level.

Quantitative assessment and determination of topography also provide evidence to throw light on the *aetiology* of the deficiency and this is of capital importance from the therapeutic point of view.

In addition to the topographical aspects of the deficiency which show the site of the lesion and enable a distinction to be drawn between root and trunk damage, some morphological anomalies in the potentials provide further diagnostic evidence. This is the case with traces consisting of high-amplitude polyphasic potentials frequently encountered in damage to nerve roots.

This information is particularly valuable in closed injuries and would merit further attention if it were not beyond the scope of this paper.

However, from the prognostic point of view, the most important contribution of the EMG in determining nerve trunk lesions lies in the possibility it gives to differentiate between transient crushing and long-lasting physiological division (with or without loss of continuity).

When a nerve trunk is sectioned, spontaneous fibrillatory activity consisting of small short-lived potentials appears in the days following the accident. This change corresponds to spontaneous activity of the striped muscle fibres of the motor unit, which have been isolated from neuronal control. It reaches its peak in the third week, when Wallerian degeneration has become established and remains at that peak as long as the degeneration lasts.

In the case of physiological section, i.e durable loss of conduction but without any anatomical gap, as occurs in compression by a fracture, the persistence of the factor responsible for the deficiency results in an EMG pattern identical with that of an anatomical gap, and they cannot be differentiated by electrical means. However, it is relatively uncommon in the case of a loss of conduction without section, not to see some active motor units and this, despite everything, makes it possible to discard the assumption of total section.

On the other hand, in the case of crushing of a nerve trunk leading only to transient loss of conduction, the spontaneous fibrillatory activity is weak and sometimes completely absent, or else from the very first weeks there is a tendency for the muscle fibres to become resynchronized. This is a reassuring picture which justifies a certain optimism, particularly if these favourable factors are confirmed by subsequent examinations.

Thus, from the diagnostic point of view electromyography of a damaged nerve provides positive topographic and biological evidence which cannot be neglected in already closed lesions or even less in partial sections, in which clinical diagnosis proves to be more difficult and where sometimes indications for resection of a partial neuroma may arise.

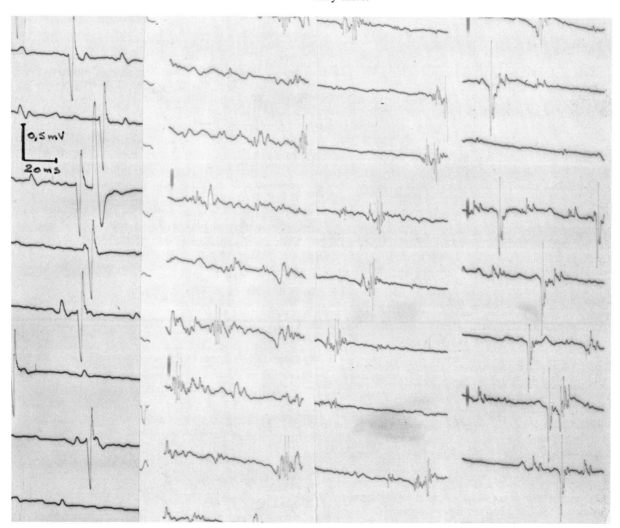

Figure 4.1
A, normal action potential
B, 25-year-old adult

Extensor Carpi Ulnaris: small polyphasic reinnervation potentials 8 months after repair of section of the radial nerve in the arm.
C, D, Hypothenar Muscles: reinnervation potentials 10 months after section and repair of the ulnar nerve at the wrist.

PROGNOSTIC VALUE

When a total nerve section has been diagnosed and repaired, the EMG can still provide useful information for establishing a prognosis.

The time which elapses before the first clinical signs of regeneration can be seen is particularly long and electromyography will often provide information earlier. Furthermore, while the appearance of Tinel's sign shows a favourable prognosis, the increase in formication is not always followed by motor recovery, which is an essential element in regeneration.

Electromyography has the advantage of demonstrating, long before the first clinically detectable sign of voluntary muscular contraction, sometimes over two months earlier, the electrical activity of a few motor units, thus providing evidence that some axons have recovered their power of conduction.

In many cases Tinel's sign is still a long way ahead and from the clinical point of view not the least voluntary muscular contraction can be observed.

This recovery of voluntary activity should be very carefully investigated and requires thorough exploration millimetre by millimetre of the body of the muscle. This sometimes requires the placing of a dozen or so electrodes in order to be able to identify a motor unit. Sonic detection of the motor unit is done at a distance. The sound is used to guide the movements of the electrode and to find the position which will give the best picture of the potential.

This study of potentials proves essential, for in addition to the recovery of some motor units a very favourable prognostic factor lies in the appearance of the low voltage and jagged traces and, above all, in the morphology of the action potentials which are polyphasic with small grouped potentials, spread out and of low amplitude. This pattern, which corresponds to a resynchronization of the denervation potentials, demonstrates that re-innervation is in progress and provides evidence that recovery will continue. Indeed, these so-called re-innervation potentials change with the progress of recovery of the nerves. They are gradually modified during recovery and progress little by little towards normal morphology. Their presence shows that further progress is still possible and that it would be premature to have recourse to surgical stabilization.

The problem is not so simple in the case of partial lesions. The active motor units which are identified may be connected with axons not affected by the lesion. Furthermore, the morphological anomalies in the potentials which reveal progressive neurogenous damage, may equally well be a sign of a deficiency which is regressing, or of gradual aggravation of the lesion through ischaemic disorders or partial neuroma. In this case a comparative examination carried out six to eight weeks later confirms whether regression or exacerbation is taking place by showing whether the trace is richer or poorer in potentials.

A proviso must be entered as to the prognostic value of electromyography. While it shows that a deficiency is regressing and that recovery is progressing it is nevertheless impossible to forsee the final extent of recovery and whether progress will not stop somewhere along the way, and whether important disabilities will persist or not.

From the point of view of prognosis, electromyography provides valuable information, since it precedes the clinical signs of recovery and shows that progress is under way and will continue. However, it is impossible by means of electromyography to forsee the extent of ultimate disability. It is only through repeated examinations that the moment will be detected when re-innervation has ceased to progress, leaving surgical stabilization as the only possibility.

Electromyography, then, proves useful in practice:

1. In the diagnosis either of a lesion which clinically is difficult to interpret, or the provision of medico-legal confirmation before surgical intervention.
2. To formulate at an earlier stage following repair a prognosis in regard to recovery and decide whether to allow re-innervation to proceed or to proceed to surgical stabilization.

5. NEUROGRAPHY IN LESIONS OF THE PERIPHERAL NERVES

J. P. Razemon, B. Petyt and G. Bonte

Neurography consists in radiological demonstration of the nerve trunks with positive contrast medium. It is applied to traumatic lesions of the nerves, external compression, and internal lesions.

It is indicated in two types of lesion:

In paralysis of traumatic origin, particularly of the upper limbs, in which the nerve was not explored at the outset. The injury present is examined at the stage of stabilized disability and the problem is to find out whether the nerve is in continuity or divided, whether there is a regeneration neuroma, or if, where there is no visible gap in continuity, there is physiological interruption of the nerve.

Neurography, after clinical and electrical tests, has provided us with valuable additional information.

In paralysis arising in cases where there has been no injury, whether accompanied or not by a palpable tumour, and suggesting external compression or a lesion of the nerve itself.

DEVELOPMENT OF THE TECHNIQUE

It was following work in particular by researchers on leprosy at Dakar that we thought that this technique of examination might be applied to traumatic lesions of the peripheral nerves.

In 1948 Vilanova and Steller carried out the first neurographies, using Thorotrast but without satisfactory results, it seems.

In 1965 Carayon published the results of twelve neurographies in cases of leprotic neuritis. He used ultrafluid Lipiodol either by injection through the skin or by exposing the nerve over a short distance.

In the same year Cave published the results of 100 neurographies of the ulnar nerve in persons with leprosy, still using ultrafluid Lipiodol.

These two latter authors emphasized the diagnostic and prognostic value of neurographic examination in cases of leprosy. They noted no complications during these examinations but pointed out that the product persists for two or three weeks before being resorbed.

In 1969 Bassett presented six cases of ulnar neurography.

He emphasized that in addition to leprosy, which undoubtedly required a neurographic examination with Lipiodol, the technique was of great value in the aetiological diagnosis of familial ulceration of the extremities and in the topographical diagnosis of nerve tumours. He pointed out that the ease with which the examination could be made and the perfect toleration of the contrast medium make it possible to use this type of examination, without risk, to supplement the usual clinical and electrical diagnostic tests.

In 1969 Gaujoux described a case of external compression of the median nerve discovered after injection of Duroliopaque.

Since all these authors emphasize that the nerve showed full tolerance to the contrast medium, we felt able to apply this exploratory technique to lesions of the peripheral nerves.

TECHNIQUE

In cases of leprosy, neurographic studies were most often carried out percutaneously, since they involved large nerve trunks, easy to find and puncture.

In case of traumatic lesions of the nerves we decided to make a surgical approach to the nerve a dozen centimetres above or below the lesion, the area to be explored depending on the clinical signs. Once the nerve had been exposed it was punctured with a fine catheter. Only one puncture was made so as not to destroy the neurilemma and not to cause leaks which would falsify the radiological pattern and prevent the injection of an adequate amount of the medium. In any case, such leaks are difficult to avoid completely and during the injection it is necessary to sponge away very gently the excess of liquid which may escape from the nerve.

The catheter is connected to a low-pressure syringe and we inject 3 to 4 ml of Duroliopaque. The injection must be made slowly over an average period of 20 to 30 minutes. It has seemed to us that the contrast medium moves better when the injection is made under the neurilemma at very low pressure rather than in the central part of the nerve.

The progress of the contrast medium is followed using an image intensifier.

During the injection the nerve is seen to swell slightly. The injection must be sufficiently slow to avoid any burst of the neurilemma and we prefer to supervise this with the naked eye. At the outset we thought it would be simpler to close the wound up again as soon as the puncture was made and to withdraw the catheter later when the liquid had all been injected, but we preferred to dispense with this technique and the wound is, therefore, closed up at the end of the operation.

We chose ethylmonoiodostearate, or Duroliopaque, which had already been used by Gaujoux. It is indeed the most fluid of the iodized oily products. Its iodine content is 29 per cent and its viscosity 28 centipoises. Its molecule is comparable to that of Lipiodol etc., its main characteristic being, as we have already stated, its low viscosity.

This product is currently used in positive-contrast myelography without having any toxic effect on the nerve roots which lie inside the dura mater. It is also used in epidurography and diffuses partly along the elements of the lumbar plexus without giving rise to any particular trouble.

It is valuable for the topographic diagnosis of the lesion to be made during the injection. Indeed, the contrast medium normally tends to diffuse along the healthy portion of the nerve and it will make very little spontaneous progress towards the nerve lesion.

Radiographs are taken during and at the end of the injection and within 48 hours following the examination in order to determine precisely the appearance of the lesions observed.

We have thus carried out 15 neurographs for paralysis of nerve trunks in the upper limbs, one for the sciatic nerve and one for familial ulceration of the extremities. We have seen no secondary complication and no change in the normal recovery following reparative surgery of the nerve.

Failures of the method were due, once to the fact that we used a water-soluble product, twice because of injections made so far away from the lesion that it was not reached by the contrast medium, and once when exploring a lesion situated below the carpal tunnel.

NORMAL NEUROGRAPHIC APPEARANCE

After injection the nerve shows a regular diameter, decreasing gradually from the root of the limb to its end. A characteristic fasciculated appearance can be distinguished and the medium moves into the collateral branches.

When the nerve is free the medium diffuses in a few hours along the nerve trunk, which shows a regular appearance.

Whatever the direction of the injection it has become obvious that the limits of exploration in the upper limbs are represented at the top end by the brachial plexus,

which we have never managed to inject by this method, and below by the carpal tunnel, which represents an anatomical obstacle which can be passed only under pressure.

We have been struck by the fact that even in cases of efferent injection the contrast medium has a tendency to move up rather than down along the nerve sheath. That is why as far as possible we believe that it is useful to make the injection below the site of the clinically suspected lesion.

COMPLETE SECTION OF THE NERVE

The complete section of a nerve is marked by arrest of the flow of the contrast medium. Near the point of section there is often a leak, as if the pressure were becoming too great. Furthermore, the nerve is enlarged and loses its fasciculated appearance over a certain distance (a few millimetres to a centimetre). It is probably that at this point there is a mass of fibrous tissue and that during reparative surgery over this distance there must either be frank resection of the segment involved or fascicular neurolysis.

THE CASE OF D.E.S.

This man was hospitalised for ulnar paralysis, which had occurred after an injury by a cutting instrument on the anterior surface of the forearm.

He showed an ulnar claw-hand accompanied by paralysis of the interossei with complete anaesthesia of the inner border of the hand. There was a positive Froment's sign.

Neurography showed a total arrest of the movement of the contrast medium, where the nerve became enlarged and lost is fasciculated appearance.

The surgical exploration showed complete section of the ulnar nerve (Fig. 5.1).

THE CASE OF D.U.B.

Following injury to the lower extremity of the right forearm, paralysis in the territory of the median nerve was noted.

Neurography showed that the contrast medium stopped 1 cm above the inferior radio-ulnar joint. There the nerve was enlarged and had lost its fasciculated appearance; there was a leak of the contrast medium.

Surgical exploration showed complete section of the median nerve (Fig. 5.2).

NEUROMA

When a bulky neuroma has developed at the proximal end of the nerve its neurographic appearance is quite clearcut. It shows the nerve enlarged like the clapper of a bell. The picture is quite clear at the beginning of the injection but quickly becomes vague as a result of the frequent and often considerable leaks of the contrast medium.

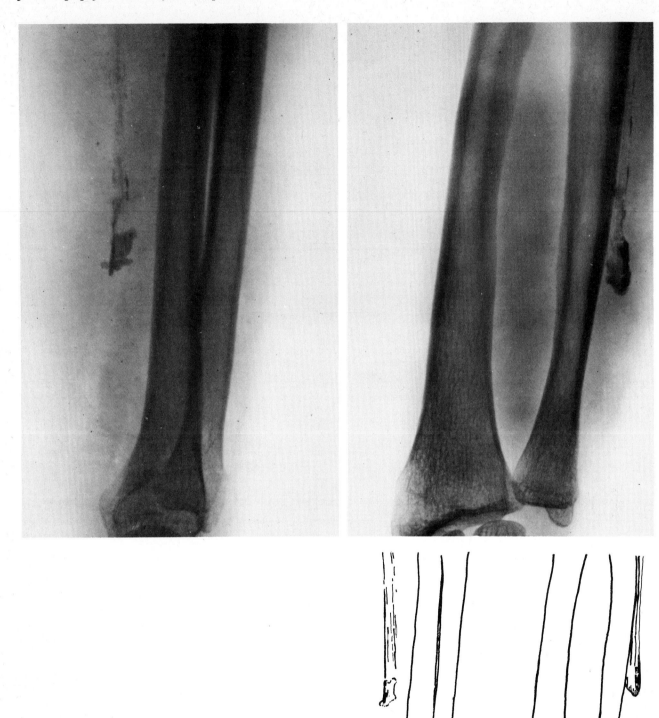

Figure 5.1
Complete section of the ulnar nerve in the lower third of the forearm. Neurography was carried out by injection about 10 cm above the lesion. Its fasciculated appearance can be clearly seen in the normal part of the nerve. Where the lesion begins, the advance of the contrast medium has stopped and the nerve is enlarged and has lost its fasciculated appearance.

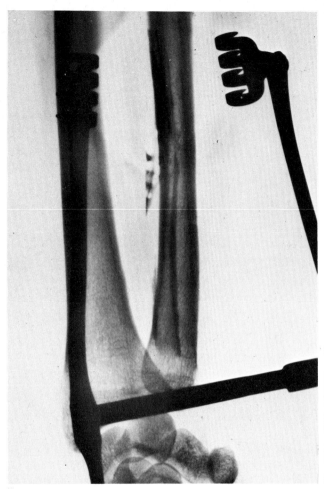

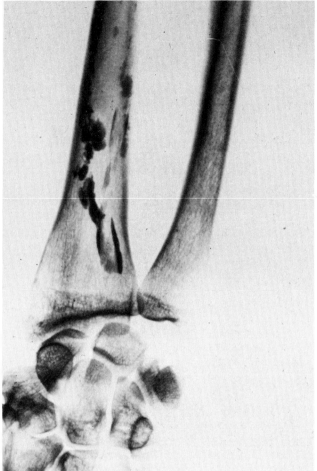

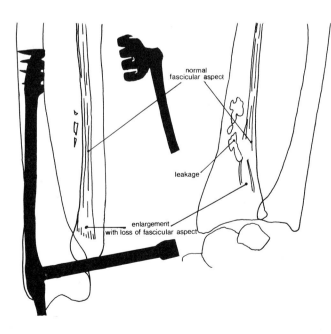

Figure 5.2
Complete section of the median nerve above the wrist. Neurography shows stoppage of advance of the contrast medium, enlargement of the nerve, the loss of its fasciculated appearance and a leak of the contrast medium. Surgery confirmed that the nerve had been completely sectioned.

THE CASE OF C.H.R.

Following a fall an injury to the anterior surface of the forearm was sutured without the nerve being examined. The flexor carpi ulnaris tendon was sutured with steel wire.

Six months later the patient was seen with a serious ulnar paralysis with sensory disorders and considerable motor disturbances accompanied by wasting of the adductor pollicis and of the whole of the hypothenar eminence. The two medial fingers were clawed.

Electrical examination showed total deficiency of the interossei and an 80 per cent deficiency of the hypothenars. Neurography showed complete stoppage of the contrast medium 2 cm above the inferior radio-ulnar joint opposite the tendon suture wires, which were visible. The nerve was enlarged; the picture showed an oval, amorphous gap. There was a leak of contrast medium later on, 4 hours after the injection (Fig. 5.3).

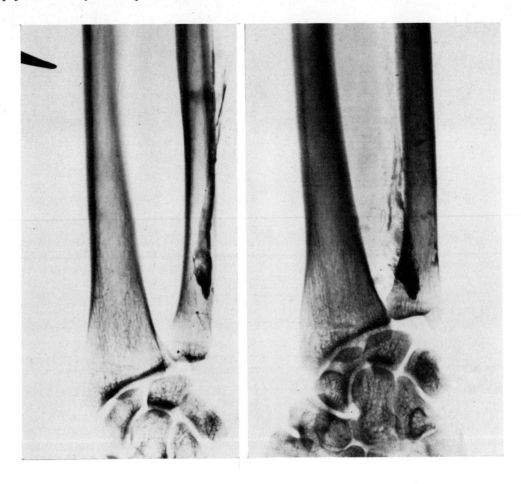

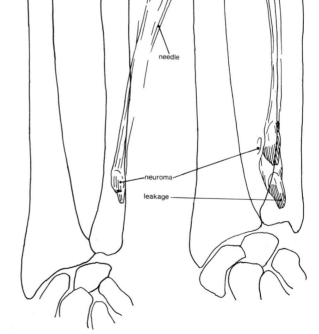

Figure 5.3
The first X-ray was taken during the injection. The needle is *in situ* 8 cm above the lesion. The appearance of the neuroma is particularly clear, with enlargement of the nerve and loss of its fasciculated appearance. Moreover, fragments of the steel wire which was used for a tendon suture can be seen. The first surgeon had missed the lesion of the ulnar nerve, and following the appearance of signs of ulnar paralysis, neurography was carried out before surgical exploration. The second radiograph, taken 4 hours after neurography, shows a leakage of the contrast medium.

When surgery was carried out (Figs. 5.4, 5.5) a nerve was found in which the neuroma and glioma were separated by a few millimetres. After resection the nerve was sutured.

Sensory and motor recovery was remarkable and seems not to have been influenced by the presence of the contrast medium.

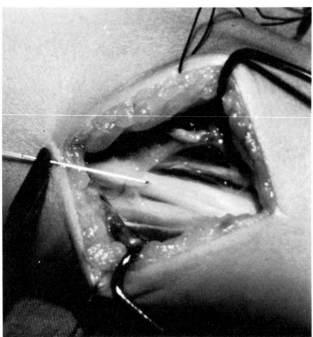

Figure 5.4
Same case as in Figure 3.1. Photograph taken at the beginning of neurography. The ulnar nerve has been uncovered and preparations are being made to puncture it, taking care to make only one perforation and to keep the needle under the neurilemma.

EXTERNAL COMPRESSION

Passage of the contrast medium through a normal channel (carpal tunnel, Guyon's canal and the canal between the olecranon process and the medial condyle) holds up its advance a little but the nerve retains its normal diameter. When there is frank compression the nerve is slightly enlarged above the obstacle and the fact that it is compressed is shown by considerable delay in the flow of the fluid, to the extent that it may be thought to have stopped. However, radiographs taken 24 and 48 hours after the exploration show that the medium had passed and prove that the nerve had not been sectioned.

THE CASE OF R.O.E.

The patient, a 35-year-old man, examined for ulnar paralysis in the left arm 4 months after an injury to the elbow accompanied by a comminuted fracture of the olecranon, showed an ulnar claw-hand and Froment's sign accompanied by wasting of the interossei and paralysis of the adductor pollicis.

Electrical tests had shown signs of partial peripheral denervation in the territory of the ulnar nerve.

Neurography showed a slowing-down in the advance of the contrast medium together with enlargement of the ulner nerve in the segment between the olecranon and the medial condyle by external compression. A leak of the contrast medium probably corresponded to a collateral branch. This was confirmed during the operation, in which the nerve was found to be intact but compressed. The ulnar nerve was transposed in front of the medial epicondyle.

The case progressed favourably, as shown by electrical examinations (Fig. 5.6).

Figure 5.5
Same case as in Figs. 6.3, 6.4. Photograph taken during the surgical repair of the nerve.

The neuroma, which is clearly visible on the right, is separated by a few millimetres from the distal glioma. The small tract which seems to join the two extremities contains no nerve fibres. It explains, however, the fact that the lesion was subtotal at the outset and appeared to the first surgeon to be relatively superficial. The neuroma and glioma, however, remained sufficiently close to each other to enable direct suture under the microscope after they had been resected.

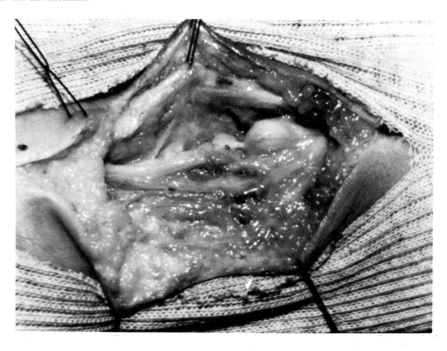

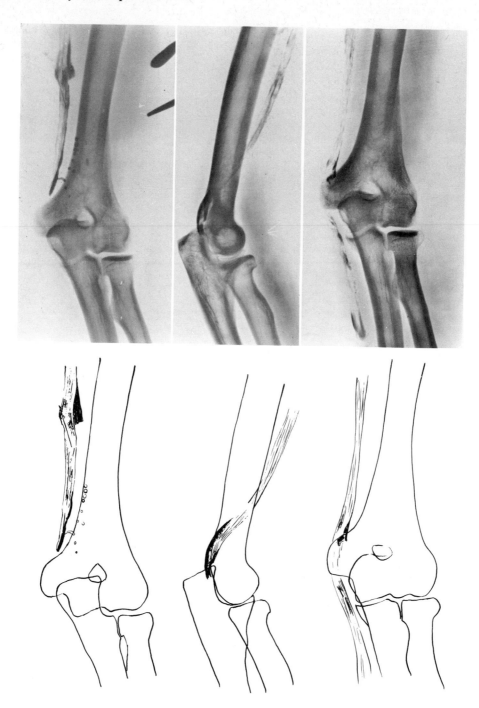

Figure 5.6
Ulnar paralysis 4 months after an elbow injury with comminuted fracture of the olecranon.

The first neurography was taken during the injection. It shows a slowing-down of the contrast medium. In the supra-epicondylar region there is a leakage which indicates an obstacle to the advance of the medium.

The second picture, taken 1 hour after injection, shows that the medium has scarcely made any progress. There is very clearly a retraction of the nerve at the entrance to the passage between the medial condyle and the olecranon.

The third picture was taken 24 hours later. The medium has passed towards the distal part of the nerve. Compression is marked and is shown by an enlargement of the nerve above the passage and very poor visibility of the nerve in the passage itself. However, the fact that the medium has progressed to the forearm shows that the nerve is not sectioned and this was confirmed during the surgical exploration, which showed a nerve engulfed by fibrous tissue. The nerve was released and transposed in front of the medial epicondyle.

THE CASE OF X

A 35-year-old woman patient was suffering from ulnar paralysis, which was ascribed to a tumour at the base of the hypothenar eminence.

The problem was whether it was a neuroma or a tumour of another kind which was compressing the nerve.

Neurography showed that the contrast medium found difficulty in advancing when faced with the anatomical obstacle represented by Guyon's canal. The medium then crossed the canal and the internal sheath of the nerve was seen to be laminated, which is a sign of external compression. The tumour was punctured and the contrast medium injected showed the presence of a cyst at the base of the hypothenar. Surgical exposure pinpointed the cyst as the cause of compression.

Other patterns can certainly be brought to light but we have not been able to work in a sufficiently accurate manner to provide valid descriptions.

This was the case with neurography of a sutured nerve in which the suture was a success, with motor and sensory recovery. It would be interesting to know whether the contrast medium crossed the inevitable obstacle formed by the suture plane and if so, to what extent.

Finally, the most interesting pattern will be that of a nerve seemingly continuous to the naked eye but in which a diaphragm of connective tissue is preventing any nerve impulse from passing. Such cases can be seen either after injuries where scar formation has induced considerable proliferation of connective tissue or after a nerve suture done under poor conditions with inadequate resection of the fibrous scars formed by the glioma and the neuroma. In such cases, in the course of a second operation, it is very difficult to decide, even under the microscope, between frank resection of the pathological zone followed by repair through suture or graft, and a simple or intrafascicular neurolysis.

The 18 neurographies we have carried out so far have not yet enabled us to find patterns characteristic of such lesions. Further work will perhaps enable us to provide some interesting information on this subject.

CONCLUSION

Our experience is still too recent for us to estimate the value and precise importance of neurography as part of the exploration of lesions after injury. It is only after a larger number of studies that we should be able to present a pattern of signs which, we feel, should be more varied than the mere arrest of the advance of the contrast medium.

In complete sections of nerve, in addition to the stoppage of the contrast medium, we have been struck by the enlargement of the sheath, which seems empty over the last centimetre, and the loss of its fasciculated appearance. In this case, therefore, we see an area which will probably have to be resected during surgery and it was valuable to obtain this information.

In external compression, with an enlarged laminated nerve, the site, extent and repercussions of the compression on the nerve are shown up clearly by neurography.

Neuroma demonstration seems to us to be characteristic.

Finally, neurography seems to us to be the most suitable technique for the discovery of tumours of the main nerve trunks and Bassett[1] has published an account of a benign Schwann-cell tumour of the ulnar nerve which was shown up perfectly by neurography.

We have been unable so far to find any characteristic appearance of a sutured nerve or of an anatomically continuous nerve which is physiologically interrupted. It is, however, along these lines that, as a supplement to the obvious and important information provided by electromyography, neurography can usefully contribute to the pre-surgical tests to be carried out in lesions of the peripheral nerves.

6. FROMENT'S SIGN*

Jacques Roullet

Froment's sign, the classical sign of ulnar nerve paralysis, was reported to the Neurological Society of Paris on 7 October 1915.

Being privileged to have in my possession a manuscript of Jules Froment's, dealing with the thumb adduction sign, I thought it might be valuable to restate the main points in the development of the symptom and the reflections it inspired in me.

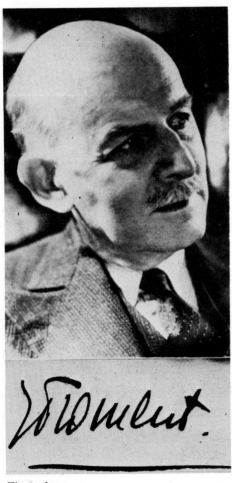

Figure 6.1

At the very beginning of the First World War, Jules Froment, Professeur Agrégé and Médecin des Hopitaux in Lyons, was mobilized with the rank of Medical Officer, Second Class. His duties gave him the opportunity of working in Paris in Babinski's Department at the Pitié Hospital. The research carried out by these two distinguished neurologists led to the emergence of a memorable description of the symptomatology of motor paralyses on the one hand, and hysteria, pithiatism and nervous troubles of reflex origin on the other. The number of wounded and persons suffering from nervous diseases coming from the front explains the preoccupations of these two research workers, the direction in which they pursued their investigations and the abundance of clinical facts they observed.

What was known of the part played by the adductor pollicis in grasping during these first few years of the First World War? Duchenne of Boulogne, through his experiments with the topical application of electricity, had provided a remarkable description of the facts. His ideas are scrupulously reported in Jules Froment's manuscript:

The adductor pollicis and the deep portion of the flexor pollicis brevis draw the first metacarpal towards the second and move it forwards and a little outwards. The first metacarpal moves in different directions, depending on the position it occupies when contraction takes place.

The adductor pollicis and the deep portion of the flexor pollicis brevis flex the first phalanx, bend it back on its inner border and impart to it a movement of rotation on its longitudinal axis in the opposite direction to that produced by the abductor pollicis brevis and the superficial portion of the flexor pollicis brevis.

Finally, the adductor extends the distal phalanx of the thumb like the extensor pollicis longus and the abductor pollicis brevis.

These ideas call for some comment.

* Work done at the Orthopaedic Surgery Department, Lyons. Director of the Clinic: A. Trillat.

37

Figure 6.2
The two basic types of pinch grip:

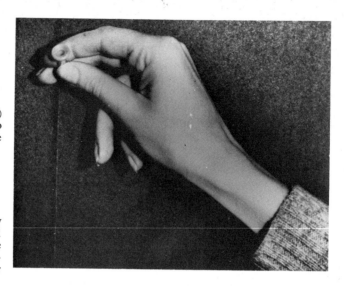

A, The pollicibidigital pinch or three-jaw chuck (precision grip) Note the fundamental role of the thumb which is brought into opposition (antepulsion and pronation) by the action of the muscles of the thenar eminence supplied by the median nerve.

B, The pollicilateral digital pinch (power pinch) demonstrated by the 'sign of newspaper' (Froment's sign). Note the fundamental role of the thumb in powerful retropulsion as it clamps over the supporting column provided by the flexed fingers. This retropulsion is produced by the adductor of the thumb supplied by the ulnar nerve.

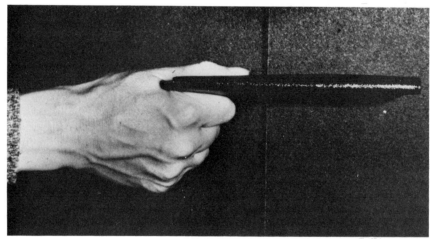

We have not attempted stimulation of the adductor but in a case of isolated traumatic paralysis of the thenar ramus of the median we saw what amounted to confirmation.

On the healthy side the grasping of a small object resulted from a harmonious pincer movement which brought the mechanism of opposition into play: the thumb and the index finger, their pads touching, formed a circle.

On the injured side, in grasping the same small object, the ulnar border of the thumb was pressed firmly against the radial border of the index. The pad of the thumb was 'apposed' against the lateral surface of the nail of the index finger. The muscles of the first interspace become very protruberant and this demonstrates the lack of proportion in the power of this grasping movement. This posture arises from laterodigital prehension. The adductor, the deep portion of the flexor pollicis brevis, and the first dorsal interosseous muscle alone come into play.

What part is played by the adductor and the deep portion of the flexor pollicis brevis in the movement which brings

the pad of the thumb beyond the median axis of the hand towards the base of the little finger?

Jules Froment, in the preface to the paper he read to the Neurological Society, had pointed out that the adductor could only bring the thumb to brush the palmar surface of the hand at the level of the first and second digital radii: beyond that, in the direction of the little finger the opponens muscles took over, the thumb went into pronation and moved gradually away from the plane of the palm.

This same patient, suffering from isolated section of the thenar ramus of the median nerve, enabled us to verify this notion.

On the intact side, the thumb easily reached the basal flexure crease of the little finger, passing over the axis of the third radius in an elegant movement of circumduction.

On the paralyzed side, the thumb, when pressed hard against the second and third ray, had difficulty in reaching the base of the ring finger.

The adductor is therefore essentially a powerful agent

for adduction of the thumb against the palmar surface of the radial border of the index and middle fingers, whatever the starting position.

Duchenne, having seen a case of isolated paralysis of the adductor pollicis, had noted that the main uses of the hand were preserved and that the patient could write, but the hand felt too tired to hold a pen for any length of time and the patient only had a weak grip on objects put in his hand. This was all that emerged at that time from the symptomatic description of ulnar nerve paralysis, alone with sensory disorders and the claw-hand syndrome.

Jules Froment, in a summary table of the disorders resulting from ulnar nerve paralysis of the muscles of the thumb, had stated under the heading of adductor and flexor brevis that it was impossible to bring the thumb and its metacarpal up to the index finger, which always remained separated from them at the base.

However, on his manuscript, written in a different ink, is the note 'incorrect'.

This correction was certainly made at the same time as the description of the thumb adduction sign and is justified

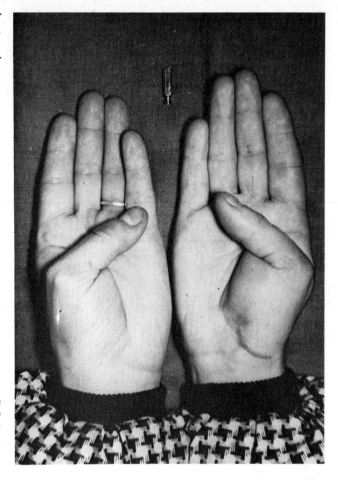

Figure 6.3
Effects of an isolated division of the thenar motor branch of the median nerve only, *sensibility being normal* in the median territory. A, On the patient's right hand, a curved scar can be seen on the lower part of the thenar eminence. The patient has been asked to bring the pulp of the thumb across to touch the lower part of the little finger on both sides. Note that on the right injured hand the anteposition-pronation of the thumb is absent. The thumb is not able to go further than the fourth ray.

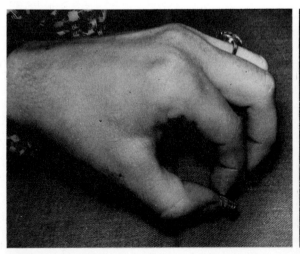 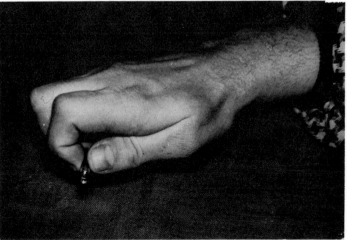

B, With the normal hand, the patient is able to pick up a small object, with a precision pinch consisting mostly of anteposition and pronation of the thumb, due to the action of the opponens and short abductor supplied by the median nerve.
C, On the injured side, the attitude is different. As the opponens and short abductor are paralysed, picking up a small object between the thumb and the index is produced by a substitution of actions. The thumb moves into retroposition, demonstrating very well the strong retropulsive action of the adductor, supplied by the ulnar nerve.

by a passage in the original communication to the Neurological Society which states that, despite paralysis of the adductor, the thumb can generally still be pressed against the index finger, although in every case it is found that in doing so the distal phalanx is flexed. Froment commented that this was a substitution due to the synergistic action of the flexor and extensor muscles of the thumb.

The adduction component of the extensor pollicis longus muscle is well known. It is due to the angulation of the extensor pollicis longus around Lister's tubercle on the lower end of the radius. It can easily be demonstrated in total poliomyelitic loss of the intrinsic muscles, in the course of which the thumb is cocked back behind the metacarpal plane. In this very special substitution movement, as Boyes pointed out, flexion of the thumb has the effect of bringing the long extensor tendon under tension in such a way that the whole power of the muscle is exerted on its adductor component.

To determine whether the adductor and the deep part of the flexor brevis were intact or disabled, an everyday automatic action had to be found which involved simultaneous execution of the various tasks performed by these muscles; deficient adduction of the thumb was not the objective.

The familiar gesture with which we seize hold of an object between the thumb and the index finger, particularly when the object is thin, fulfils all these requirements.

In practice, as Jules Froment taught, a folded newspaper should simply be held out to the patient, who is asked to grasp it successively with his intact and his damaged hand, while quite strong traction is being exerted.

On the healthy side, the thumb presses hard along its whole length against the object grasped, and the distal phalanx is completely relaxed or only very slightly flexed. This is the normal, standard energetic grasping movement, effected by contraction of the adductor.

On the paralysed side, the thumb strains, brings the distal phalanx into strong flexion and, whatever strength is exerted, only the tip of the pulp presses against the object. In most cases there is a real gap between the thumb and the newspaper. Finally, but how obvious this is varies in different cases, a movement of opposition is not present, but the thumb is turning outwards and moving away from the metacarpophalangeal articulation of the index.

This was the 'newspaper sign' Froment described, but how did he interpret it?

The patient brings into play the system for grasping with the thumb which is usually kept for delicate prehensile movements. The prehensile posture is the work of the opponens muscle and the adductor brevis, and the strength of the pincer movement is due to the contraction of the flexor pollicis longus.

It is very important to note at this point that this substitution of movements is altogether different from that observed in cases of *total* loss of the thumb muscles, when substitution brings only the extensor pollicis longus and the flexor pollicis longus into action.

In Volume VI of the neurological section of Sergent's Treatise on Medical Pathology, Jules Froment wrote the chapter on paralysis of the motor nerves. He added to the description of the 'newspaper sign' the various gestures of everyday life which primarily bring into action the adductor pollicis.

In cases of ulnar nerve paralysis, he indicates that the patient finds it difficult to turn a key if the lock is stiff, that the shoemaker or saddle-maker finds it difficult to handle his paring knife, that the coachman experiences some difficulty in holding the reins and that tailors find it hard to use the needle. What remains topical nowadays is the picking-up of a knife, which it is impossible to do normally in cases of ulnar nerve paralysis. In one of the striking phrases for which he had a flair, Jules Froment said that to remedy this state of affairs the patient would have to seize his knife with his hand 'as if he wished to carve up a side of beef'.

Is it possible from this interpretation of the part played by the adductor pollicis in the gestures of everyday life to draw any indication as how to treat paralysis of the adductor?

While the synergistic action of the extensor longus and the flexor muscles of the thumb makes it possible to alleviate the absence of adduction of the thumb, the laterodigital pincer movement which this substitution brings into play is nevertheless inadequate.

Recourse to fine pincer movements is more logical, since in the normal state they can be powerful, but in the case of adductor paralysis the 'newspaper sign' demonstrates that the substitution is inadequate: despite the strength of the flexor muscles of the fingers, the thumb slips.

The 'newspaper sign' shows that the proximal phalanx of the thumb is placed in extension at the metacarpophalangeal joint and has a tendency to turn outwards towards the radial edge.

We consider that the precariousness of this fine pincer movement, which is substituted for the laterodigital pincer movement in cases of adductor paralysis, can be ascribed to the instability of the metacarpophalangeal joint on its ulnar margin.

To alleviate this instability it is not so much a question of restoring the powerful adduction of the thumb as of balancing the proximal phalanx of the thumb by means of a graft on its ulnar margin.

In Professor Merle d'Aubigne's Department, Raoul Tubiana recommends the grafting of the flexor superficialis, reflected around the superficial palmar aponeurosis, directly to the ulnar margin of the proximal phalanx.

Boyes, whatever the method chosen, recommends that an available interosseous space should be used as a pulley mechanism. He prefers to keep tendon transfers as a means of compensating for the absence of the adductor in cases of combined paralysis of the median and ulnar nerves.

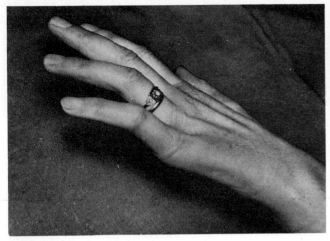
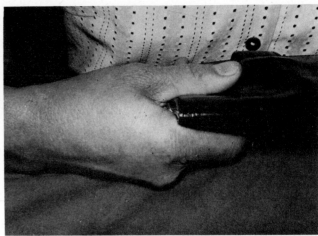

Figure 6.4
Paralysis of the Ulnar Nerve
A, Low paralysis of the ulnar nerve, typical begging attitude (only a moderate degree of claw hand in this case).
B, Testing of the pollicilateral digital pinch power grasp by Froment's sign on the healthy side. The thumb in retroposition, with slight flexion of the proximal phalanx, is clasped above the clenched fingers. The flexor pollicis longus is not contributing. The first dorsal interosseous is seen to contract strongly in the first interosseous space.

C, On the side with ulnar paralysis, the same attempt leads to a different attitude because adductor power is absent from the thumb which is unable to move into retroposition. The thumb attempts to grasp the object with anteposition, hyperextension of the MP joint and flexion of the distal joint. This substitution involves first the short abductor of the thumb in the three-jaws pinch movement. Thus there is seen anteposition and a tendency to pronation, and introducing the action of the flexor pollicis longus provides increased power. The first dorsal interosseous does not work and the first interosseous space is seen to be hollow. The grip is unstable if there is antagonist traction the object will slip out leaving an aperture in the web space between the thumb, the index finger and the object. This demonstrates the Froments' 'newspaper sign' when there is an ulnar paralysis.

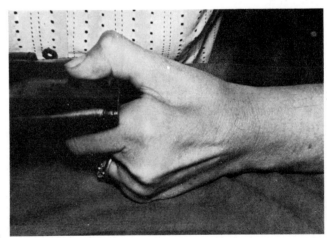

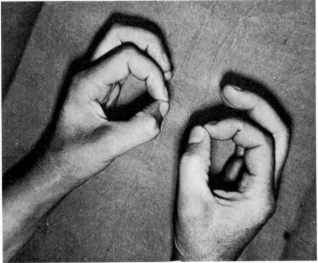

D, Another case of ulnar paralysis in the left side showing that the pinch appears normal because the median nerve is intact. Of course in this motion the atrophy of the first interosseous space is seen, and in order to demonstrate the ulnar nerve lesion it is essential to search for the 'newspaper sign'.

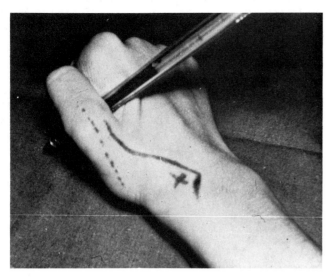

Figure 6.5
Paralysis of all the intrinsic muscles of the thumb after poly-myelitis, showing the substitution of movements used by the patient for writing, and demonstrating the complementary retropulsive action of the extensor pollicis longus. This substitution of motion which involves for one part the extensor pollicis longus with its retropulsive component and also the flexor pollicis longus, has nothing in common with the previous substitutions observed either in isolated ulnar paralysis or isolated median paralysis.

It appears that indications should be rather wider, judging from the satisfaction of the patients in whom such grafts have been carried out.

CONCLUSION

According to the definition given by Babinski, the term 'objective sign' is reserved solely for a really conclusive sign that a normal man, however clever and knowledgeable he may be, cannot imitate exactly.

The 'newspaper sign' which is a classical sign of ulnar nerve paralysis, meets this definition and, to the analysis of the abnormal grasping motion which it indicates, should be added the finding that there is no contraction of the first dorsal interosseous muscle.

From the point of view of the prognosis, the 'newspaper sign', better than any electrical examination, enables us to follow recovery from ulnar nerve paralysis. Indeed, the gap which appears between the thumb and the lateral margin of the index grows gradually smaller as the nerve recovers.

The 'newspaper sign' is an excellent test for assessing the effectiveness of palliative muscle grafts in cases of adductor paralysis. Grafting proves effective when it modifies Froment's sign in the sense that the thumb slips less and the proximal phalanx is slightly flexed and no longer turns outwards towards the radial margin.

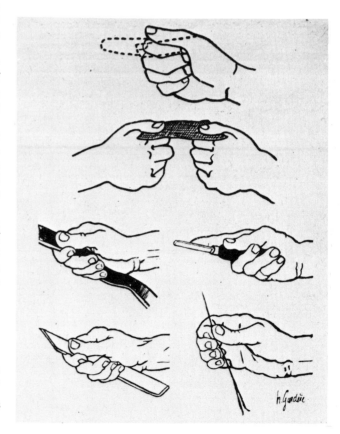

Figure 6.6
Document illustrating the 'newspaper sign' taken out of the historical publication by Jules Froment in '*La paralysie des nerfs moteurs*', Paris Maloine et Fils, 1924

The adductor of the thumb, its action and the different types of grip depending on it.

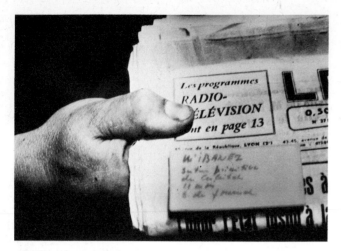

Figure 6.7
Froment's 'sign of the newspaper' is not only a test for diagnosis but also a test for assessment in relation to surgery.

A, Eleven months after suture of the ulnar nerve, the 'newspaper sign' has improved in that the grip has become stable and there is no more gap in the web space between the thumb and the index finger. Note the visible first dorsal-interosseous appears in the first space.

However, the flexor pollicis longus still plays its part, and the first dorsal interosseous is not quite as firm as normal on palpation. Froment's sign has therefore the value of a quantitative test to which could be added, either the measuring of the surface of the first web space gap, or a dynamometric test to study the progress of stability of the grip.

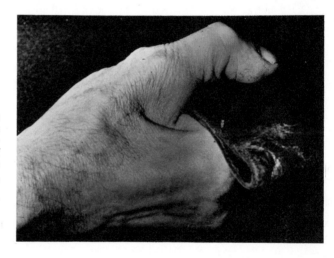

B, Ulnar paralysis after transfer of extensor proprius into the insertion of the adductor pollicis through the second interosseous space. This transfer is required to stabilize the metacarpophalangeal joint on its ulnar side. It is of course the instability of the ulnar side of the MP joint which is basically responsible for the attitude of substitution of the power pinch in ulnar paralysis, that is, for Froment's sign.

One year after the operation, the substitution attitude can be seen with the changes that occurred as the grip improved and stabilized. Note only a slight flexion at the metacarpophalangeal joint and the disappearance of the web aperture.

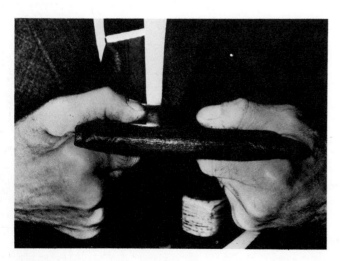

C, Stabilization on its ulnar side by tendon transfer to the metacarpophalangeal joint in ulnar paralysis, now seems well enough established to become a formal indication for improving prehension in these patients.

We usually transfer a flexor digitorum sublimus to the ulnar side after passing it through the second interosseous space. It thus approaches the thumb on the dorsal aspect of the first interosseous space.

7. *EVALUATION OF AN ACUTE TRAUMATIC PERIPHERAL NERVE INJURY*

George E. Omer

The principles for initial management of a severe extremity injury have been well established. A clean wound, structural alignment, and prevention of deformity are all important goals. Recovery of muscle-tendon activity and restoration of sensation are required for a functional hand. A peripheral nerve injury presents problems in evaluation, repair, and substitution.

EVALUATION AT THE TIME OF INJURY

Initial examination establishes the diagnosis and is a baseline against which can be noted progressive sensory or motor loss due to haemorrhage or oedema. Ischaemic injury is always pertinent during fracture manipulation or circular plaster immobilization.

The autonomous sensory zones for the three major nerves can be tested by delicate pinprick. Deep or heavy pressure may be positive, even when the nerve is completely severed. The autonomous zone for the median nerve is the volar surface of the terminal two phalanges of the index finger and terminal phalanx of the long finger. The ulnar nerve has autonomous supply over the volar middle and distal phalanges of the little finger. Radial nerve loss produces an inconstant zone of sensory deficit over the first dorsal interosseous muscle.

Evaluation of motor function should report the level of injury and the quality of motor activity. The examiner should concentrate not only on the digital motion but on the muscle producing it. Palpate the muscle belly and tendon. If possible, the muscle should function against gravity. One should be aware of mechanical advantage movements, such as passive dorsal extension of the wrist from active flexion of the fingers. Double or atypical innervation is common in the intrinsic muscles of the hand and accurate evaluation demands meticulous examination. The abductor pollicis brevis muscle has the most reliable median innervation of the thenar muscles. The ulnar nerve supplies both the abductor digiti quinti and the first dorsal interosseous. The radial nerve supplies the extensor pollicis longus, which can be tested with the extended thumb gesture of the hitch-hiker. Unless the patient fully extends the wrist and then fully extends the fingers against gravity the examiner cannot be sure that the extended digits are due to ulnar innervated intrinsic muscles instead of the radial innervated extensor digitorum communis.

Loss of sweating should parallel sensory loss and examination of the involved finger tip with an ophthalmoscope will demonstrate beads of perspiration in the uncooperative patient.

PERIODIC FOLLOW-UP EVALUATION

Many nerve lesions are not seen on the day of injury by the attending surgeon, and are neither evident lacerations nor obvious missile disruptions. The neuropathy may be secondary to oedema and reactive fibrosis which will subside in time. These patients need evaluation by multiple quantitative tests that are repeated at regular intervals. Comparison of these tests series determines the need for surgery or provides the evidence of nerve recovery. We performed approximately 15,000 separate tests in the series of periodic studies for more than 750 patients at Brooke General Hospital between January 1966 and July 1968.

SENSORY TESTS

Each point on the skin has multiple innervation and there are no morphologically specific nerve terminals in the human serving *only* warmth, cold, touch or pain. The tests with cotton-wool and pins for touch and pain and the ordinary test-tube contact for testing warmth and cold are unsatisfactory for estimating functional loss and are impossible to duplicate periodically in quantitative terms. These studies demonstrate only protective sensation.

We use the technique of marking off the hand into seven zones (Fig. 7.1). Testing is begun at the more sensitive pulp tip (Zone 7) and is continued proximally—either all the way proximal on each digit or all across the hand at each level.

In 1894, von Frey attempted to standardize stimuli by testing the subjective sensation of touch with a series of horse hairs of graduated force. We use the Weinstein and Semmes calibrated nylon monofilaments. The patient's hand is placed comfortably on a flat surface and care is

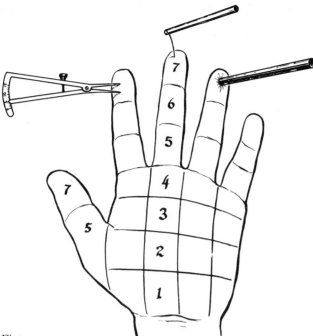

Figure 7.1
The band zones for testing sensation. The creases for the interphalangeal joints, the interdigital skin web, and the palmar creases are utilized for drawing these lines. The von Frey test tends to demonstrate returning sensation before the Weber test; while the Weber test gives the more critical reading.

TABLE I   Forces exerted by the monofilaments used in measuring sensory thresholds (milligrams)

Sensation	Fingertip	Thumb	Palm
Normal	2·36–2·83	2·44–2·83	2·44–2·83
Diminished	3·22–3·61	3·22–3·61	3·22–3·84
Protective	3·84–4·17	3·84–4·17	4·07–4·31
Loss of Protective	4·31–6·65	4·31–6·65	4·56–6·65

taken not to stimulate the proprioceptive fibres within the deeper tissues, either by small joint movement or stretching pressure. The filament force is exerted perpendicular to the skin surface and is continued until the filament bends. The hand is touched with the lighter filaments first. The patient's eyes are closed and, if he feels the filament, he opens his eyes and localizes the spot touched with a small wooden dowel the size of an ordinary lead pencil. If he does not cover the precise indentation point where the hair touched the skin, it is considered negative. If the patient misses the same weight twice in the same skin zone, a new filament of heavier force is selected. Room temperature should be even, since humidity affects the stiffness of the nylon filaments.

On occasion, the patient will miss the indentation point in a zone, but will precisely cover that same point when the next more proximal zone is stimulated. This summation usually happens just before protective sensation is regained (Fig. 7.1).

Testing of two-point discrimination was introduced by Weber in 1835 and involves touching of the skin with one or two blunt points. The points are applied simultaneously with minimal pressure and the line between the points is longitudinal to the finger (Fig. 7.1). The patient's eyes are closed. The distance between the points is varied and the patient immediately states whether he feels one or two points. In each finger zone, three tests are performed in variation—a single point is touched and two points are touched twice. If the patient does not record two of the three correct, it is considered a failure at that distance. The normal threshold for the volar surface is shown in Table 2. The threshold of the dorsal surface is generally higher. It is between 5 and 20 millimeters from the distal tips to the proximal part of the hand.

We have done approximately 1700 von Frey and 1700 Weber tests at Brooke General Hospital during the study period.* These sensory tests are really subjective and of little value in the very young or uncooperative patient.

SYMPATHETIC INNERVATION TESTS†

Only the proximal portion of the brachial plexus, central to the level at which sympathetic fibres enter, can be injured without damaging corresponding sudomotor function. Minor developed the iodine-starch test in 1928. The ninhydrin printing test was developed by Oden and von Hofsten and made practical for routine clinical studies by Moberg. We have performed 1278 sweat tests by placing the entire patient in a dry heat box and then a solution of 25 per cent cobalt chloride in 99 per cent alcohol is painted on the hand, and perspiration changes the solution from blue to pink colour. The result is recorded by photographing and drawing the hand.

ELECTRICAL DIAGNOSTIC STUDIES‡

In 1907, Peterson and Jung observed changes in the resistance of the skin to the passage of electrical current during a period of emotional change. This finding was utilized by Richter to develop a dermometer. The resistance is increased when the current encounters a dry, unsweating surface. This method is useful in the uncooperative patient.

An interrupted (indirect, alternating, faradic) current is used to stimulate the motor nerve. If the muscle contracts, the nerve is intact. Wallerian degeneration may not be complete before 21 days and response may be falsely positive during this period.

* These tests were performed under the supervision of Major Janet L. Werner, A.M.S.C., U.S.A., Assistant Chief, Occupational Therapy Section, Brooke General Hospital.

† These studies, including muscle testing and electrical diagnostic tests, were performed under the supervision of Lieutenant Colonel Rachel Adams, A.M.S.C., U.S.A., Chief, Physical Therapy Section, Brooke General Hospital.

‡ These tests were performed under the supervision of Captain Sarah D. Lopez, A.M.S.C., U.S.A., Physical Therapist, Brooke General Hospital.

TABLE 2 Return of two-point discrimination (thirty digital nerves)

2 PD	Neg.	20–16	15–11	10–7	6 mm or less
No. of nerves	3	1	3	12	11
Length of the grafts					
2 cm	2	—	1	4	5
3 cm	1	—	—	2	1
4 cm	—	—	—	—	2
6 cm	—	1	2	3	3
8 cm	—	—	—	3	3

In 1868, Erb described the response of normal and denervated muscles to electrical stimulation. A quantitative study can be done by electrical stimulation of varying strength and duration (the strength–duration curve). Normal muscle responds to an electrical impulse with a brisk twitch and prompt relaxation. The denervated muscles require a stronger current when stimuli of short duration are employed. If the muscle response is plotted on a semilogarithmic graph, it is characterized by shift of the strength–duration curve upward and to the right. If there is re-innervation of the muscle, the curve flattens and shifts to the left.

A normal muscle requires little current to contract it and much current to tetanize it. The galvanic–tetanus ratio is sometimes used as the degree of muscle denervation. It is defined as a minimal uninterrupted (direct, galvanic) current required to produce a 1 second sustained contraction (tetany), divided by the strength of current required for a threshold contraction (twitch rheobase). In normally innervated muscle, this ratio may be 1:6 or 7 but, in denervated muscle, the ratio approaches 1:1. The galvanic–tetanus ratio was evaluated over a 1 year period in ninety-six patients at Brooke General Hospital. Thirty-nine muscles showed clinical evidence of re-innervation during this investigation, utilizing a current duration of 1 second. Twenty-seven of the thirty-nine had a ratio of 1:1·5, or greater, which was a prognostic accuracy of 69 per cent. In a second clinical series, involving more than 600 patients, the galvanic–tetanus ratio predicted the clinical outcome in more cases than either chronaxie or the strength–duration curve.

Electromyography is an almost esoteric means of assessing muscle activity but is an excellent tool for the experienced. We have performed this study in 1278 instances for 677 patients from January 1966 through July 1968.* A normal muscle is electrically silent at rest and, when it contracts, motor unit action potentials are recorded. When a muscle is denervated, the silence is replaced by many small deflections called fibrillation action potentials (fibrillation or denervation). Attempts at voluntary contradiction do not change the electrical pattern. Fibrillation is not an im-

mediate property of denervated muscle but usually occurs 2 to 3 weeks following the injury. However, we have noted fibrillation action potentials 1 week following severe nerve lesions, such as a phosphorus burn wound. We mistrust electromyography 6 months or more after nerve injury. The electrical study is reporting a small muscle mass instead of the total muscle, and may show return of activity that will not result in clinical function.

Helmholtz measured the conduction velocity in the human median nerve in 1852, with results about the same as current findings. Nerve conduction time is particularly valuable in anatomical localization of a nerve injury.

However, the investigator must consider mechanisms other than injury that may decrease the velocity of nerve conduction. Examples would include alcoholic, diabetic, or nutritional polyneuropathies. In addition, there are yet unresolved questions concerning speed of conduction in relation to the strength of stimulus, the size of the nerve fibre, and the age of the patient Grioce Otis found to decline after 30 years of age (Table 3).

TABLE 3 Motor nerve conduction—normal values (milliseconds)

	Time Wrist latency	Rate Conduction Velocity
Ulnar	2·7 (1·6–4·1)	59·1 (49·1–65·5)
Median	3·4 (2·4–4·6)	58·5 (47·0–64·3)
Radial	5·8 (4·2–7·1)	56·3 (48·0–64·0)

VOLUNTARY MUSCLE TESTING

Voluntary muscle testing establishes the exact level of active and inactive muscles and probably is the best available for the surgeon. However, the examiner should be aware that the patient is a sophisticate in 'trick movements', particularly about the thumb, about 6 months after injury. Voluntary muscle testing should be repeated at regular intervals of 6 to 10 weeks. In addition, the quality of contraction needs evaluation so that serial studies can be compared.

Highet's Clinical Scale:
    0—total paralysis
    1—muscle flicker
    2—muscle contraction
    3—contraction against gravity
    4—contraction against gravity and resistance
    5—normal

* The electromyography and conduction velocity tests in this study were performed by Lieutenant Colonel Walter H. Moore, Jr., Medical Corps, U.S.A., Chief, Physical Medicine Service, Brooke General Hospital.

Every time the voluntary muscle test is performed, all the pertinent muscles in the extremity should be examined. An adequate list would include:

Ulnar nerve
    Flexor carpi ulnaris
    Flexor digitorum profundus (little)
    Abductor digiti quinti
    Adductor pollicis
    First dorsal interosseous
Median nerve
    Flexor carpi radialis
    Flexor digitorum profundus (index)
    Flexor pollicis longus
    Flexor digitorum sublimis
    Abductor pollicis brevis
Radial nerve
    Triceps
    Brachioradialis
    Extensor carpi radialis (both)
    Extensor digitorum communis
    Extensor pollicis longus
    Extensor indicis proprius

FUNCTIONAL TESTS

These are the most important tests for effective study. Hand grip can be measured in pounds. We utilize the gross grip of the uninjured hand as the standard for the injured hand, with the non-dominant hand gripping 10 to 15 pounds less than the dominant hand. If both are injured, we consider a normal between 90 to 100 pounds. Functional activity of grip can be evaluated by grasping smooth wooden tubes of varied diameter. Finger pinch is also measured in pounds, both tip (5 to 10 pounds) and lateral (Key) (13 to 20 lbs). In the very weak hand, Swanson places a rolled tourniquet inflated to one hundred millimeters of mercury. The patient's grip can be measured then in increased tourniquet pressure.

Moberg's pick-up test measures tactile gnosis and is measured by the time required to pick up nine objects of different size and shape. The injured hand is again checked against the uninjured hand; but, a normal in our test is 5 to 8 seconds.

The surgeon can check the course of his treatment periodically by measuring the volume displacement of the hand. If dependency or excessive activity have increased oedema, the hand will displace additional water in the volumetric test.

VALUE OF PERIODIC EVALUATION

These series of tests are of little value as individual studies. They must be repeated at regular intervals between 6 and 10 weeks to chart the continuing status of the injured nerve. They are quantitative tests that can be studied by colleagues, ancillary personnel, and the patient, himself. Only precise studies accurately reflect the progress of treatment.

If the sixteen tests we use are repeated every 6 weeks, the patient's records will contain sixty-four separate tests after six months. To correlate these findings, a hand packet has been developed on our service to collect and demonstrate the trend of the multiple tests.* We find multiple periodic tests most valuable in the obscure neuropathy that is seen late in the course of treatment, or is neither an evident laceration nor obvious missile disruption. Testing at regular intervals until 6 months after injury will demonstrate those three out of four injuries of this type that will return to clinical function. All tests should be used in problem cases; but, after reviewing our 15,000 tests in more than 750 patients, we believe a minimum battery would include: two-point over autonomous zones; sweat test; galvanic–tetanus ratio; voluntary muscle study with recorded range of motion; and a timed pick-up test.

INTERVAL REHABILITATION

From the time of injury, the hand is kept in a dynamic functional position. The principle of active motion of scarred muscles cannot be neglected and daily activities should be emphasized. This requires a team approach which includes: occupational therapist, physical therapist, splint maker, as well as a cooperative patient and an interested surgeon.

A most important aspect of treatment is the need for individualized dynamic splints, which should be made for each patient and then adjusted whenever indicated. Problem areas have been maintenance of the transverse palmar arch and of the thenar web space, adequate lumbrical and thenar stops for position, and excessive tissue tension from traction.

FACTORS INFLUENCING NERVE REPAIR

There are indications for both primary and delayed repair of nerve injuries. Everyone develops a set of manifestos based on his own failures: (1) don't perform a primary repair of a major nerve disrupted by a gunshot wound; (2) if debridement exposes the nerve and judgement decides against repair, the nerve ends can be tagged with fine wire to prevent retraction and for roentgenological identification; (3) extensive elective incisions are unnecessary and may be harmful. If the nerve is freed completely from its soft tissue bed over many centimeters, its blood supply is in jeopardy. All above-elbow ulnar nerve

* The hand packet was developed by Major George G. Rakolta, Medical Corps, U.S.A., Orthopaedic Service, Brooke General Hospital.

Rakolta, G. G.

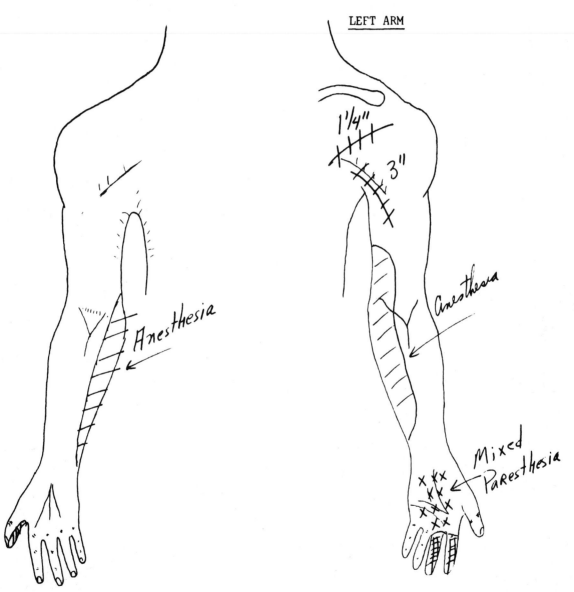

Figure 7.2
Outline sketch of upper extremity. Here is recorded the location of wounds, operative incisions, fractures, and sensory changes of the extremity. The reverse side shows the contralateral extremity.

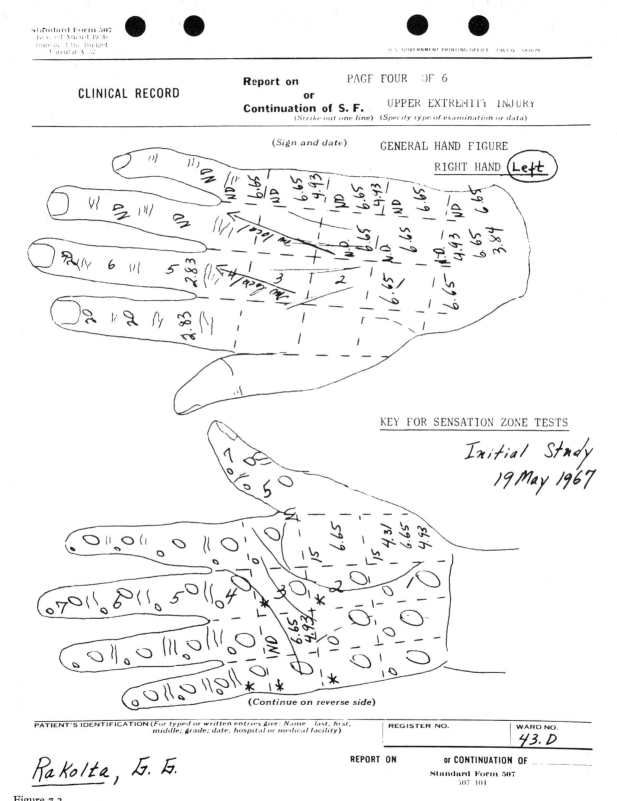

Figure 7.3
The key for the sensory zones and an outline sketch for location of injury involving the hand. The reverse side shows the contralateral extremity.

repairs with associated anterior transplants of the ulnar nerve at the elbow have had poor results; (4) optical magnification will make nerve suture technically easier; (5) as small a non-reactive suture as compatible with the mechanics of the repair should be used. We use 6-0 stay sutures, with 9-0 and 10-0 monofilament nylon (Ethicon) for the repair; (6) there should be minimal handling of the nerve during repair; (7) there should be minimal tension on the suture line—failures have been reported with only 5 per cent stretch. Occasionally, the fibrous outer shell of the neuroma can be step-cut and these longer tongues sutured along one side of the nerve repair to relieve total tissue tension; (8) the repaired nerve should be placed in a bed of healthy soft tissue; (9) the skeleton should be stable to prevent excessive callus entrapment or movement at the nerve suture line. However, immediate metallic fixation of the fracture in a severe injury invites osteomyelitis; (10) time after anastomosis must be a factor in the results. Functional return for a peripheral nerve is 1 millimetre per day, or approximately the length of a phalanx per month. The ulnar nerve has a tendency to be much slower to recover functionally than the radial or median nerves, and this should be considered before undertaking muscle-tendon transfers for ulnar deficiency.

The technique of multiple nerve tests at regular intervals should be continued after surgical repair. Gradual return of function may be demonstrated and relieve apprehension but testing will also indicate the need for re-suture or muscle-tendon transfers.

8. THE EFFECT OF TRAINING ON SENSORY FUNCTION

Edward E. Almquist

It is becoming increasingly apparent that the specific modality tests of von Frey do not give a sufficient estimate of cutaneous sensory function. The best quantitative measure of return of sensory function of the hand after nerve suture has been shown to be two-point discrimination. These results correlate with tactile gnosis, the term used to describe the ability of the skin to identify objects by touch. One, therefore, tends to substitute two-point discrimination values for tactile gnosis, since the latter itself defies measurement. A question, then, may arise as to whether tactile gnosis or two-point discrimination is a fixed value not possible to improve beyond a given limit and depending on the anatomy of the nervous system, or whether tactile gnosis can be improved by training.

Probably the best possible example of training would be found in blind people who read Braille very rapidly. These readers identify letters by patterns of small round raised mounds, punched in paper. These mounds are 1 millimetre in diameter and separated by 1 millimetre.

Eleven blind rapid Braille readers were tested for two-point discrimination and compared with a normal individual for age, sex, texture of skin, and ability to co-operate and concentrate. Their ages were from 20 to 58 with an average of 41.7 years; five were males and six were females.

A compass was used as an instrument for stimulus. The points had been blunted to a surface of 0.25 millimetres. This was enough to produce a small stimulus by pressure, but not to produce pain. The patients were seated comfortably and their dominant hand was allowed to assume a relaxed position while their arm rested on a pillow. The hand was then held firmly in this position by resting the dorsal side on a solid object and fixing the fingernail with the examiner's own nail. The fingers were in moderate flexion. Originally complete extension was used, but it became obvious that more consistent readings were obtained with the hand in a resting position. The stimulus was applied rapidly to the finger with just enough pressure to give a very small, blanching effect adjacent to the points of the compass. The stimulus was at right angles to the skin. Almost invariably the best results for two-point discrimination were obtained when the points were perpendicular to the skin rugae. The two-point skin stimulus was measured, not by distance between the stimuli, but the distance between the outside margins of the compass.

Originally it was thought that the Probit method of analysis would be used to determine the two point distance. In this the number of correct two-point determinations would be subtracted from the number of incorrect one point stimuli and the two-point distance was taken when the 50 per cent value was reached. It became obvious, however, that there was a sharp demarcation between the distance when one and two points could be resolved. If the examiner was careful and the examinee was comfortable and relaxed, essentially 100 per cent values could be obtained when testing the two-point distance within a very narrow distance; therefore this absolute value was taken. The reading finger was used for the analysis and this finger invariably had the best two-point discrimination. The controls were tested in exactly the same manner and the dominant finger with the best two-point discrimination was recorded. Usually, but not always, this was the index finger. No patient with a known medical illness or previous hand injury was used. People who were anxious, in a hurry, or for other reasons could not cooperate were not used.

RESULTS

The eleven blind Braille readers had an average two-point distance of 1.31 millimetres. The range was from 0.75 to 2.25 millimetres; there was a sharply demarcated distance where these patients could resolve two from one point (Fig. 8.1). The control group had a range from 2.75 to 4.25 millimeters, the average distance was 3.34 millimeters. This distance is highly significant with a P value equal to 0.00049 with the Sign test. The demarcation also was quite distinct between the distance when one and two points could be resolved, but the control people would often not answer as quickly after a stimulus application as the Braille readers. It was, however, impossible to quantitate this observation.

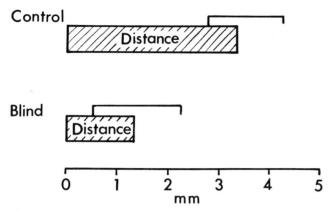

Figure 8.1
Method used for two-point discrimination test with control and eleven blind subjects.

DISCUSSION

The fact is shown that, with appropriate training, a remarkable degree of tactile sensory function can be obtained. This then would suggest that the limit of sensory resolution is dependent on the brain's interpretation of stimulus received from the skin. Certainly it is reasonable to assume that the anatomy of the sensory neurons or nerve endings is no different in the blind than in normal people.

A mechanical stimulus is recorded by a nerve ending for a considerable distance away from the stimulus and not as von Frey suggested, just by the sensory receptor directly beneath the stimuli. This can be demonstrated by stimulating an insensitive area of fresh, thick skin graft or in an area of surgical denervation. The stimuli are received depending on closeness to the sensible skin nerve or nerve endings and on the amount of pressure. More pressure will depress the skin for a greater distance and hence stimulate receptors further away. This would suggest therefore, that the nerve electric mechanism for transmission of two-point discrimination is based on a spatial pattern of stimuli recorded on the skin and sent to the central nervous system, and not on two neurons each sending its separate message to a cortical level. The resolution of the pattern between one and two points is at least in part a central nervous system function that can be affected by training.

SUMMARY

Eleven Braille readers were subjected to a two-point discrimination test to quantitate the degree of acuity in their reading fingers. Their resolution of sensibility was significantly greater than similarly tested controls. It is suggested that the greater degree of sensibility results from the ability of the central nervous system to learn to resolve smaller spacial patterns of sensory stimuli.

9. PHYSIOTHERAPY AND FUNCTIONAL REHABILITATION AFTER LESIONS OF THE PERIPHERAL NERVES

Georges H. Fallet

INTRODUCTION

Of the three basic and now classical types of nerve lesion defined by Seddon, which are, in order of severity, *neuropraxia*, *axonotmesis* and *neurotmesis*, only the physical treatment and functional re-education required by the two last will be considered in this paper. Neuropraxia, in which the axons remain intact results only in a short-lived interruption of nerve conduction, so that the loss of sensory and motor function which accompanies it will regress in a few weeks without any need for serious therapeutic measures. The case is quite different with axonotmesis and neurotmesis, where severe disorders follow which are often partially or totally irreversible and the sequelae of which will certainly be more serious if a suitable programme of physiotherapy is not planned.

In some circumstances the nature of the injury and the operative findings will leave no doubt as to the anatomical type of nerve lesion involved. Very often, on the other hand, and all the more so if surgical exploration has not seemed necessary straight away, it will be impossible, despite the most refined electrodiagnostic examinations, to determine at the outset with any real certainty, whether axonotmesis or neurotmesis is involved, or as often occurs a combination of the two types of lesion. Indeed, in axonotmesis and neurotmesis the initial clinical and electrical signs are identical.

However, the differential diagnosis between these two conditions is of prime importance. With axonotmesis there is justification for anticipating spontaneous regeneration of the nerve fibres in a normal anatomical way, whereas the total gap in continuity left by neurotmesis will require surgical suture of the two ends of the nerve, without which any regenerative process would be impossible. Furthermore, the process may be less perfect since each proximal fibre will not necessarily find again that distal fragment which was originally connected to it.

In both cases, regeneration of the axons and the myelin sheath will require considerable time the length of which depends to a great extent on the latent period before the process begins (about 30 days), on the distance between the site of the lesion and the muscles dependent on the part of the nerve which has been damaged (the average speed of regeneration of a nerve fibre is roughly 1 mm per day) and in the case of a suture the time which elapses between the injury and the surgical procedure.

During all this time, which will often amount to a number of months, it is essential to apply a programme of physiotherapeutic measures to the totally or partially paralysed limb first of all for preventive purposes and then for gradual re-education in order to achieve at the end of it all the best possible functional results (Dyer, Wynn-Parry, Yeoman). Some of these measures, however, are tedious and should only be undertaken when there exists a real possibility of recovery; they are illogical and superfluous when the lesion present is permanent.

This paper will not deal with the question of clinical diagnosis or electrical exploration nor with the surgical aspect of the treatment of lesions of the peripheral nerves and plexuses or the repercussions which these factors may have on the process of re-innervation.

It will, on the other hand, discuss which factors and consequently which physiotherapeutic procedures can influence the quality of the final functional recovery following axonotmesis or nerve suture. The programme of treatment which we apply, the various aspects of which will now be discussed, follows that now used by most departments specializing in this sphere and particularly in the Medical Rehabilitation Unit of the Royal Air Force at Chessington under the guidance of Wynn Parry, whose experience is authoritative.

FACTORS WHICH INFLUENCE RECOVERY OF FUNCTION

These are essentially as follows:
1. Oedema.
2. The condition of the skin.
3. Deformity and stiffening of the joints.
4. The motor deficiency and re-innervation potential
5. The sensory deficiency.
6. The apparatus used.
7. The intensity of the daily treatment schedule.

OEDEMA

Oedema is largely caused by the vasomotor disturbances resulting from the nerve lesion. If it persists, it may entail fibrosis of the subcutaneous tissues which may, indirectly, hinder the excursion of the muscles, tendons and joints. It is, therefore, essential to combat it from the outset by elevating the injured limb, maintaining it there uninterruptedly for a certain period; by massage, by applying bandages between every treatment session leaving the fingers or toes completely free and continuing towards the root of the limb and by applying various positional splints.

Certain types of apparatus which exert gradual and rhythmic centripetal pressure may also drain the oedema successfully (Circulator, Vasculator Jobst Bag).

CONDITION OF THE SKIN

The changes and lesions which may be seen in the cutaneous tissues result on the one hand from vasomotor disorders followed by trophic disorders of neurovegetative origin and on the other from a profound local deficiency accompanying every serious peripheral nerve lesion.

In a first stage following immediately upon the injury, the paralysis of the vasoconstrictor fibres will induce a state of congestion with hyperaemia and hyperthermia. At the end of about three weeks a second phase will ensue, during which vasoconstriction will occur, with hypothermy, a decrease and then an elimination of sweating activity and finally gradual atrophy and fibrosis of the skin and the subcutaneous tissues, which in certain cases may involve the deep tissues such as the aponeuroses, the tendons and their synovial sheaths, the ligaments, the joint capsule and even the bones. These neurotrophic changes are, therefore, liable by themselves to lead to periarticular stiffening and deformities.

Moreover the sensory deficiency in regard to the sense of touch and pain and temperature sensation associated with the vasomotor and neurotrophic disorders described above may lead to various lesions such as sloughs, burns, frostbite, infections etc., particularly if the patient's attention has not been properly drawn to these risks.

It is, therefore, important for certain measures to be instituted to prevent these complications, or at least to reduce them to a minimum, so that they do not become serious obstacles to rehabilitation. Thus an effort will be made to apply, if possible twice a day, massage with oil or talc to the skin and subcutaneous tissues, accompanied by movements of friction and circumduction at the deep levels and cautious passive stretching of the limb in order, on the one hand, to maintain the suppleness of the epidermis and dermis and, on the other, to prevent or reduce periarticular and peritendinous adhesions.

The graded application of local heat (wax baths, mud baths, etc.) will help to maintain satisfactory circulation in the superficial tissues and the muscles, making kinesitherapy more effective.

Particular care will be taken when the nails are being cleaned so as to prevent any infection.

Finally, the patient will be given precise and repeated information on the risks that he will be running as a result of the areas of anaesthesia. He will be taught to protect himself from the cold and from any source of excessive high temperature and to compensate by visual inspection, the loss of sensation of contact between the areas of the skin surface which have lost their sensitivity and the surrounding objects.

DEFORMITY AND STIFFENING OF THE JOINTS

Several types of deformity, often irreversible, may occur in the case of serious lesions of the peripheral nerves. When wounds, tendon lesions and adhesions in the limbs do not occur as complications of the nerve lesions themselves, the clinical pictures and postures which those nerve lesions bring about are perfectly well-known and characteristic. They depend on the nerve, nerves or plexus involved and the level of the lesion.

The abnormal postures and deformities which may arise are the result of several factors: the extent, distribution and severity of paralysis, the disturbed balance between certain groups of muscles (agonists and antagonists) that will occur, the musculotendinous or aponeurotic retractions present, the reactions of adhesion between the various layers of tissue, and finally articular or periarticular stiffness.

Here again, physiotherapy must have as its aim the prevention or at least the maximum possible correction of the disorders brought about by these tissue changes so that no obstacle will interfere with functional recovery at the time when the first signs of re-innervation appear. Indeed, there would be no point in having successfully sutured a radial nerve, if at the time when the extensor muscles of the wrist and fingers recovered adequate voluntary activity, they could not be used for their proper functions because of irreducible deformities such as a stiffening of the wrist in flexion or retraction of the digital flexors with their tendons and tendon sheaths in addition adhering to the palmar aponeurosis.

From the very outset, tendinous retraction of the predominant muscle groups will be combated by postural treatment, usually by means of plaster or plastic splints kept on for most of the day and night. In view of the cutaneous anaesthesia and the risk of pressure sloughing which it entails, frequent and regular inspection of the condition of the skin is essential. Serial plaster stretching splints will be all the more useful when it is a question of correcting an already existing deformity which can still be reduced without surgical intervention. The shape and angle of the splints will then be changed 'to order', often every one or two days, so as to adapt them without delay to the progress made by the physiotherapy as a whole.

Of course, these splints are removed several times a day to enable the physiotherapist or occupational therapist to apply the other therapeutic procedures prescribed, on the one hand those mentioned in the previous sections and, on the other, those which seek to maintain joint mobility by exercises which are first of all passive and then mixed active and passive if a certain degree of re-innervation is achieved. Kinesitherapy of this kind, provided that it is carried out cautiously and competently, should be undertaken as early as possible. Indeed, apart from the minimum time needed for a nerve suture line to heal, any lengthy immobilization in plaster is to be avoided, particularly if it involves distal segments of the limb away from the site of the operation or the injury. In this manner also the risk will be diminished of reflex sympathetic dystrophy developing—a relatively frequent complication whose consequences for rehabilitation are only too well-known.

MOTOR DEFICIENCY AND RE-INNERVATION POTENTIAL

Any muscle completely and permanently deprived of its innervation will undergo metabolic disturbances and histological changes which will lead finally to the total disappearance of its fibres and their replacement by functionless fibro-adipose tissue (Stillwell).

Chronological studies of such alterations show that if re-innervation occurs within 1 year, satisfactory recovery can be anticipated. On the other hand, after 3 years, in general, there is no justification for expecting a positive result unless it has been possible to slow up the process of muscular atrophy and degeneration (Stillwell).

Very rapidly, i.e. as early as 3 days after sectioning of a nerve, there is an onset of atrophy which will reach a peak at the end of 40 days and will involve an average loss of 75 per cent of the original weight of the healthy muscle (Branes *et al.*). The mechanism and intensity of this atrophy have not been explained completely. They depend on certain factors, of which the main ones seem to be lack of the neurotrophic influence exerted by normal axons on the muscle fibres, disorders of irrigation in the blood and lymph capillaries of the muscle itself, complex metabolic disturbances, probably of enzymatic origin and the regulation of which is said to depend on the intactness of the axon, excessive fatigue resulting from fibrillation, immobilization, and finally temperature, since exposure to cold accelerates the rate of atrophy (Sunderland).

When faced with complete or partial, but temporary denervation, i.e. when there are good reasons to hope that re-innervation will take place within a reasonable period of time, it is essential that every useful and effective measure possible should be taken to delay or reduce to a minimum the serious histological alterations which will occur in the paralysed muscles, so that when the moment comes, the regenerated axons will find muscle fibres and motor endplates in the best possible functional state.

The physical means used for this purpose are varied but some of them are of only very slight value.

In themselves, local application of heat, massage, and rhythmic mechanical compressions of the paralysed muscles (Wakim and Krusen) only exert a minimum and practically negligible effect. In the same way, passive kinesitherapy of the muscle groups incapable of voluntary activity, while it has the merit of maintaining joint mobility could not possibly in itself prevent or even delay atrophy.

Electrical stimulation. The muscle fibre deprived of its nerve fibre will no longer respond to excitation by faradic current but only by galvanic current. Incidentally this property is the basis for some methods of electrical diagnosis such as the strength–duration curve.

There has been a great deal of discussion on the effect of the galvanic type of stimulation on denerved muscle and it is a common practice to subject a patient suffering from paralysis following a peripheral nerve or plexus lesion to two or more daily sessions of this form of electrotherapy in the hope of avoiding irreversible alterations in the muscle fibres. However, despite varied and numerous experiments on animals and in clinical practice, unanimity on the effectiveness of this form of treatment is still remote.

In view of the importance of this aspect of treatment, it may not be without value to examine the essential reasons for the controversy between workers who are nevertheless worthy of every confidence, and if in this discussion one adopts an attitude favourable to electrical stimulation, to give details of the ways in which it can be carried out.

If after total denervation a muscle is not re-innervated, it is a known fact that at the end of 2 years it will have undergone complete fibrous degeneration, even if it has been properly treated. The question is whether there is enough evidence to justify the application of electrical stimuli to this muscle, if it can be anticipated that it will become re-innervated before that period has elapsed.

The great majority of experiments carried out in this sphere have been done on animals. It emerges from this work that electrical stimulation is capable, to a certain degree, of preventing and reducing the extent of muscular atrophy by delaying its onset and of maintaining, up to a certain level, the strength and endurance of the denerved muscle (Branes, Shaffer *et al.*, Sunderland, Wakim *et al.*). However, it seems that these observations and the data obtained from animal experiments cannot be applied to human clinical practice without further consideration.

Studies worthy of interest carried out on man are described in only a few publications. Two are essential, that of Doupe, Barnes, Kerr and that by Jackson.

The former work can be summarized as negative in its conclusions, since only treatment of an intensity greater than that which it would be possible to administer for therapeutic purposes proved capable of inducing a measurable increase in the rate of circulation in the muscles. In the opinion of these authors, conventional forms of electrical stimulation could not have any significant value in facilitating the recovery of a denerved muscle, apart from their purely mechanical effect, which is simply a means of assisting the rehabilitation exercises and conserving the mobility of the tissues. This opinion is also held by Newman and by Liu and Lewey. These latter authors consider that the beneficial effects of such treatment are not backed up by sufficiently convincing proof to justify the sacrifices in money, time, and staff which it requires.

Jackson, however, reaches positive conclusions and seems to demonstrate the effectiveness of this form of electrotherapy in regard to the metabolism of the denerved muscle. Cowman, Bauwens and Mennell are of the same opinion, although the first of these three authors draws attention to the dangers which the state of fatigue induced by the treatment may hold for the muscle fibre.

The rapidity and intensity of atrophy are highest immediately after denervation. If no galvanic treatment is applied these processes will diminish gradually in intensity but will, nevertheless, continue for about 400 days, after which the muscle volume will remain constant. When the denerved muscle is subjected to galvanic stimulation, atrophy, as measured by muscle volume or in other experiments by muscle weight, will proceed whatever happens for a relatively short period of about one or two weeks (Gutman *et al.*, Jackson, Shaffer *et al.*). On the other hand, when measured over a period extending from day o to day 100, the degree of atrophy is considerably less in electrically treated patients than in the controls. Moreover, in patients subjected to electrical stimulation the atrophy comes to an end between the 100th and 200th day. Furthermore, at least in animals, Wakim and Krusen found that galvanic stimulation appreciably improved the strength and endurance of the experimentally denerved muscle. This effect has not been verified in man.

Although galvanic electrotherapy exerts no effect on axon regeneration (Sunderland), and therefore does not reduce re-innervation time, Jackson has the impression that it contributes to obtaining better functional recovery by helping the performance of voluntary movements if it continues to be applied at the time when re-innervation is occurring (Jackson).

In children and young adults it seems that the results are in any case very much better than in older persons and that electrical stimulation is not indispensable.

Unlike Wynn-Parry, who is not convinced that galvanic stimulation has any beneficial effect and does not feel the need to have recourse to it, our attitude is that we should not deprive a patient of a form of treatment which even if it is not certain to bring him indisputable relief could in no case be harmful to him. While applying this form of therapy we, nevertheless, remain fully aware that it is incapable of completely preventing atrophy of the denerved muscle or of preserving normal strength and endurance in such a muscle.

From the practical point of view use can be made either of square-pulse galvanic current or, and preferably, an exponential progressive current. This latter has the double advantage over the conventional square-wave stimulations of being more comfortable for the patient since the shock is less abrupt and of selectively stimulating the denerved muscle fibres while excluding those which are still intact.

This property is particularly to be appreciated when a partially denerved muscle has to be treated (Offner, Wynn-Parry).

The number of stimulations per treatment session, the size of the stimulus, and the duration and frequency of the session, are all factors which have also given rise to numerous controversies, to such an extent that at the present moment the most various opinions are still held (Stillwell, Sunderland, Wakim *et al.*). However, certain general rules emerge from these works which it is valuable to know about.

The optimum frequency of the stimuli seems to be 10–30 per minute. Each stimulus should be sufficiently intense to make the muscle work effectively, which in the opinion of certain authors means that it must contract sufficiently to develop its complete range of movement against resistance. As for the duration and frequency of the sessions, it appears that the best results are obtained by several brief applications (5 to 10 minutes) repeated throughout the day (Stillwell). A technique of this kind obviously raises practical problems which often cannot be solved unless the patient can be kept in hospital or if after discharge from hospital he does not have his own apparatus in his own home.

In our department we are generally satisfied with two sessions per day lasting 10 to 15 minutes each or with several sessions of shorter duration, to make up 60 minutes per day with intervals of rest in between.

In general, it should be recalled that a denerved muscle rapidly tires and that as a result of this state of fatigue it requires at least 10 minutes to recover (Kosman).

However, the effectiveness of electrical stimulation does not depend solely on the technical conditions but also on other factors again, such as the ambient temperature of the muscle and the size and anatomical site of the muscles to be treated. Those of smaller dimensions and nearer the surface are easier to stimulate and therefore respond best to treatment (Jackson, Sunderland).

If it is decided to apply electrical stimulation to a denerved muscle, the treatment should therefore be instituted as soon as possible after the nerve injury and be continued without interruption at suitable intensity and in adequately long and frequent sessions (Jackson, Stillwell). In view of the fact that any voluntary contraction, however small, is more effective for functional muscular recovery than the best galvanic stimulation, electrotherapy should be ceased as a rule as soon as the first clinical signs of re–innervation occur or at least soon afterwards, if it is sought to continue to facilitate the patient's efforts in this way (Sunderland).

Of course, this form of electrotherapy using other types of current may be indicated for other reasons: for example, for psychological reasons when it is a question of proving to a temporarily paralysed and discouraged patient that his muscles are still capable of functioning. In the same way a muscle transplanted for orthopaedic reasons can be successfully stimulated in order to train it for its new function by co-ordinating the electrical stimulation with active kinesi-therapy. These considerations, however, are beyond the scope of the present paper.

Kinesitherapy and motor re-education. It has been demonstrated that immobilization speeds up the mechanism of atrophy of a denerved muscle (Jackson). It is, therefore, of the highest importance, even in the case of complete paralysis, that the muscle or muscle groups involved should be passively mobilized.

As soon as the first clinical manifestations of re-innervation appear, the patient's co-operation will be sought in order to exploit to the utmost every effort of voluntary contraction. First of all, use will be made of active and passive exercises in the ordinary way or in a swimming pool, followed as progress in functional recovery occurs, by free active exercises, and finally by exercises against increasing resistance.

Since we have to deal with lesions of the peripheral motor neuron, it is possible to apply the classical techniques of rehabilitation and muscle-building (Gardiner), based on the principles laid down by de Lorme, taking care by calculating maximum resistance and gradually regulating the number of exercises per session and the frequency of the session to increase simultaneously the strength and the endurance of the muscle. These methods, of which several variations exist, are now too well-known for detailed description to be necessary.

It goes without saying that the latest techniques of motor rehabilitation, derived from various neurophysiological principles of neuromuscular facilitation and inhibition and some of which are based on schedules of over-all movements, also occupy an important place in the physiotherapy of the sequelae of lesions to the peripheral nerves and plexus (Gardiner, Kabat, Knott, Voss).

Finally, occupational therapy, with its infinite variety of ingenious methods, will also play a predominant role in the schedule of treatment at all stages of evolution.

Whatever the methods used, progress will be periodically assessed by means of electrodiagnostic checks and above all, with greater simplicity, by manual tests based on the criteria laid down by Lovett and then by the British Medical Research Council. The codes in this system which range from o (complete paralysis) to 5 (normal muscle) make it possible to estimate quite accurately and more or less quantitatively the strength of each muscle or group of muscles. This method of evaluation is indeed the same as that which we use for diagnostic purposes (Daniels).

SENSORY LOSS

Any severe lesion of a peripheral nerve entails in addition to paralysis a more or less complete loss of the various types of sensibility in the area involved.

I mentioned above the dangers to the skin from the complete lack of protective sensibility to touch, pain, heat and cold.

Some obstacles to rehabilitation may result from the loss of proprioceptive sensation and posture sense, particularly if the nerve lesion or lesions involve the lower limbs. Re-education in walking may be delayed by this and exercises may have to be introduced for balance, co-ordination, and permanent visual checking by the patient when he moves his legs.

Finally, while it is quite common for the gross sense of touch and temperature known as the protective sense to reappear sooner or later, the patient less often recovers his capacity for fine discrimination. In cases of paralysis of the median nerve, this loss of stereognosis may be a serious handicap in daily activities and still more in professional work. Wynn Parry has developed for these cases an interesting method of re-educating sensibility. It consists mainly of training the patient to recognize objects of different shape, weight and texture, first of all blindfold and then verifying his sensations visually.

These exercises are timed, and care is taken to vary constantly the series of objects so that the patient cannot cheat by habit or using his memory. As progress is made, the diversity, size and complexity of the objects and their shapes is increased.

This technique has been in use for several years now in our occupational–therapy centre, with encouraging results.

APPARATUS

This branch of functional reeducation in the case of lesions of the peripheral nerves deserves treatment at a length which is out of the question in this paper.

In general we try to avoid any complicated and above all any static orthopaedic apparatus. When it is impossible to dispense with auxiliary means, we use for preference 'lively splints', which are extremely simple and were invented by Wynn Parry. These are easy to make and can be put together in any occupational therapy department. These splints, which are small and consequently not aesthetically displeasing, are almost always accepted by the patients. While remaining effective, they provide the maximum of freedom of movement.

INTENSITY OF THE DAILY TREATMENT SCHEDULE

Too much emphasis could never be laid on the prime influence that the daily organization of physiotherapy may exert on the standard of the final results of recovery and re-education following lesions of the peripheral plexuses and nerves. The more intense and varied the schedule, the more rapidly are functional results obtained and the better they are.

This statement has proved so true that Wynn Parry does not hesitate to bring all his cases to hospital, so that for the necessary length of time he can offer them the intensity of treatment he considers essential. It is true that his unit is subject to military regulations and that consequently it only houses injured servicemen, so that a decision of this kind is easier to take than it would be in private practice or even in civilian hospital practice.

From the outset various essential preventive measures must be put into practice, checked and repeated often in the course of the day to ensure regression of the oedema, to avoid or correct stiffening of the joints and deformities, and to delay is possible and reduce to a minimum the muscular atrophy. However, it is above all at the stage of re-innervation that the programme must be intensified and not cut down as, unfortunately, only too often happens. It is during this period that every effort must be made to use all the means at our disposal to give the muscle the benefit of the regeneration of the nerve fibres and that, where need be, any persistent sensory loss must be compensated by careful and patient re-training.

Sensory recovery and above all re-training of the strength and endurance of the muscles, which even in an athlete requires a training programme of progressive muscle-building exercises, cannot be achieved in injured muscles by means of a few exercises carried out without conviction or with no proper theoretical basis, at the rate of one or two sessions per week.

The doctor's training, the co-operation of well-trained technical staff and, above all, the motivation of the patient and his family, will all be factors which will make it easier to carry out such a programme. Very often, unfortunately, its practical implementation is hindered by simple questions of means and organization, which despite everyone's convictions and efforts find no ideal solution.

SUMMARY

Physiotherapy and functional re-education in lesions of the peripheral nerves and plexuses requires the carrying-out of various measures depending on the stage of evolution and, above all, on the re-innervation potential. Whatever else may happen, the final result of functional recovery will depend on the intensity of the daily treatment schedule.

It will be necessary from the outset to try to combat the oedema, to prevent or correct stiffening of the joints or deformities, to delay and reduce to a minimum atrophy in the paralysed muscles, and to keep those muscles in the best possible condition from the metabolic point of view while waiting for nerve regeneration to take place.

During the re-innervation phase a programme of suitably graded kinesitherapy will be undertaken in order to obtain rapid and maximum recovery of muscle strength and endurance. Progress will be detected by electrodiagnostic means or manual estimation and put in numerical form at frequent intervals, thus enabling the methods of treatment to be adjusted at any time.

Where necessary, 'lively splints' will facilitate motor re-education.

In certain cases particularly of the median nerve, it will be useful to reteach stereognosis to the best possible extent.

Whatever the stage of evolution, occupational therapy, with its great diversity of methods, must play a considerable part in the rehabilitation programme.

10. AN ELECTRICAL AND CLINICAL FOLLOW-UP OF NERVES SUTURED AT DIFFERENT AGES

Edward E. Almquist and Orvar Eeg-Olofsson

Suture of adult peripheral nerves has given relatively poor clinical results, yet nerve sutures performed in childhood usually result in an excellent restoration of function. This observation has been generally explained on the basis of a better maturation potential for children's neurons. Experimental evidence to substantiate this explanation, however, has been lacking.

This study was designed to quantitate the results of children's and adults' nerve repairs and to correlate these results with the degree of neuronal regeneration as monitored by sensory nerve conduction velocity.

Maturation of regenerated nerves was defined by Lloyd Guth as 'Those processes leading to the restoration of normal fibre diameter and normal electrical properties of the nerve'. Hursh and also Tasaki *et al.*, have shown that in normal nerves the speed of an electrical impulse along the neuron varies linearly with the nerve fibre diameter. This means that knowing the electrical velocity along a neuron, the diameter can be determined. In a series of neurons such as present in a peripheral nerve, the average diameter and the range of diameters can be obtained.

METHODS

Nineteen patients at least 5 years after nerve suture were tested by the sensory conduction velocity of the ulnar and/or median nerve at the wrist and by the two-point discrimination test (Fig. 10.1). Their ages at the time of the examination were between 10 and 35 years. At this age group nerve conduction velocity has been noted to be constant and normally the same for children and adults (Dobbelstein and Strappler, 1963; Downie, 1969; Guth, 1956; Mayer 1963). The sensory conduction velocity was performed after the method of Kemble (Mayer, 1963).

The skin temperature as measured by an Ellab thermacouple was 31–34° C.

For controls the opposite normal nerves were tested. These were monitored in exactly the same manner. Also, to assure that there was little normal variation between the conduction velocity on the right was compared with the left, the unaffected nerves were also tested on both sides. These nerves had conduction velocities of equal degree.

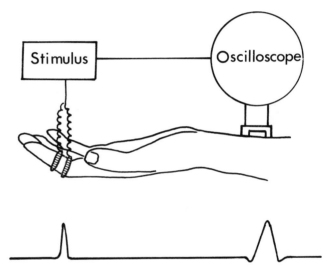

Figure 10.1
A stimulus is applied to the finger; it travels up the nerves and is recorded as it passes beneath a recording electrode at the wrist. The time that this takes divided by the distance is the conduction velocity.

Tactile gnosis is best quantitated by a meticulously performed two-point discrimination test; therefore, this parameter was taken as the most accurate measure of a degree of return of nerve function following suture (Mobena, 1958, 1962). This test was performed by the method of Önne (1962).

RESULTS

The results of the tests are shown on Figure 10.2. The control values are noted by the X markings. In these, two-point discrimination is between 2·75 and 4·25 millimeters. The nerve conduction velocity is between 48 and 70 meters per second. This velocity corresponds with the normal values obtained by others (Dobbelstein and Struppler, 1963; Downie, 1969; Gamstorp and Shelburne, 1965; Kemble and Peiris, 1967; Mayer, 1963). The data obtained from the sutured nerves are shown by dots. These nerves

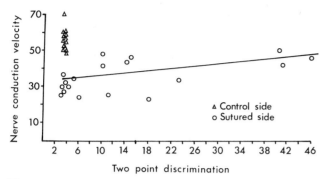

Figure 10.2
There is no correlation between the clinical result as monitored by the two-point discrimination and the nerve conduction velocity hence maturation. If there was a correlation, the curve would slope downward; the greater the slope the more direct the correlation.

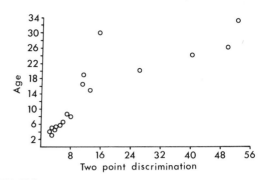

Figure 10.3
There tends to be a linear relationship between the age of the patient at the time of nerve suture and the clinical result. A patient with a nerve ideally sutured at age 5 should expect a 5 millimeter two-point discrimination and a child with a repair at age seven could expect a seven millimeter two-point discrimination and so on.

conduct between 22 and 48 metres per second. The important thing to note is that there is no correlation between the clinical results as monitored by the two-point discrimination test and the nerve conduction velocity. If there were a correlation, the curve would have turned sharply downward.

The best clinical results following surgery are all noted in children. If age at the time of suture is plotted against the two-point discrimination test, one notes that there tends to be in ideal cases a linear relationship until about the time of puberty (Fig. 10.3). The pattern after puberty tends to become more random.

DISCUSSION

This study, has confirmed that the degree of return towards normal sensation following nerve suture varies directly with the age of the patient at the time of suture (Fig. 10.4 A, B). The electrical characteristics of these sutured nerves, however, do not vary with the age of the patient. It has been shown that a patient with an excellent clinical result may have a nerve which is electrically similar to those with poor clinical results. The negative correlation between clinical results and nerve conduction velocity certainly limits the ability to use electrical values obtained on experimental animals as a means of assaying clinical results in nerve suture.

If maturation of the sutured nerve is not the important difference between the good clinical results noted in children and the poor clinical results noted in adults, what is the difference? Perhaps we can examine the factors involved in transmitting messages to the central nervous system. Neurons are the communication line between the stimulus and the interpretation centres, namely the central nervous system. Any stimulus must be expressed to the central nervous system via the neurons which are basically electrical conductors.

It then is apparent that to change the function of the

neuron as after nerve suture, the electrical properties or patterns must be changed. There are, probably four ways in which this can be accomplished: (1) a slowing or speeding of the impulse; (2) a change in the number of neuronal pathways; (3) following suture, the stimulus from a given area on the skin will eventually stimulate a cortical cell or cells in a different position than normal; and (4) the nerve endings can be altered.

With these assumptions, then, we can analyze the data and attempt to arrive at some conclusions. First, these studies have shown that the sensory conduction velocity of a sutured nerve does not positively correlate with the clinical results. Velocity change is not then the crucial factor. Secondly, there is no reason to believe that surgeons can realign a nerve of a child more adequately during repair than the nerve of an adult. Probably, in fact, it is even more difficult. Certainly then the fact that children have remarkable recovery cannot be related to the factor of alignment. Since there is no difference between good and poor results, and since nerve regrowth proceeds from proximal to distal, it would be reasonable to assume that the distal portion of a neuron (the nerve endings), would be no more mature or efficient. This leaves us with the possibility of more, yet immature neuronal pathways, as a possible difference in the sutured nerves between good and poor clinical results. Even if there were more neurons we must still presume that they have not been accurately aligned. Yet some children following nerve suture have essentially normal clinical results.

It is obvious, then that there must be another factor necessary besides the accuracy of the nerve suture to explain the difference in the clinical results. This must be the central nervous system. There is some experimental evidence to substantiate this (Benjamin). Ablation of a sensory cortex in the young as compared to the adult cats can lead to quite different clinical results. The young cat will be able to learn to differentiate sensory stimuli, the adults cannot

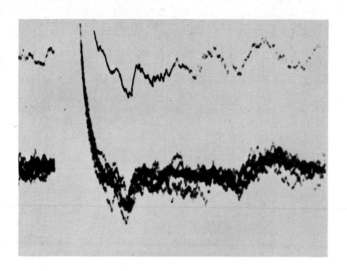 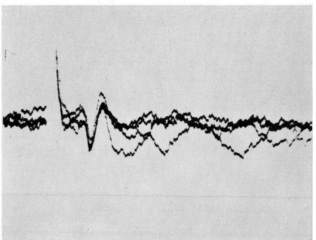

SUTURED AGE 7

Velocity = 34 m/sec
2PD = 3.75 mm

NORMAL

Velocity = 60 m/sec
2PD = 3.5 mm

Figure 10.4 A, B
These are the results in a sixteen year old male comparing the left median nerve sutured at age 7 and the normal right. Despite a very slow conduction velocity, the patient has a normal two-point discrimination.

(Benjamin). This is evidence of the adaptability of the central nervous system in young as compared to adult animals. This explanation in patients with nerve sutures would suggest that the sensory stimuli altered by the limitations of the surgical suture are learned to be correctly interpreted by the young patients' central nervous system. That is, the new clinical patterns become meaningful in children. The adults have fixed patterns and the stimuli are not properly interpreted by the central nervous system.

SUMMARY

Nineteen patients at least 5 years following nerve suture, were examined by an exacting two-point discrimination test and by a sensory nerve conduction velocity study. The conduction velocity which normally is a function of nerve diameter, did not correlate with the two-point discrimination test. Patients with very slow conducting nerves, hence small diameter neurons, may still have near normal clinical results. The clinical results as monitored by the two-point discrimination test varied linearly with the age of the patient at the time of suture until about puberty. These findings show that sensory nerve conduction velocity cannot be used to quantitate the clinical results in experimental animal studies. These findings further suggest that the adaptability of the young patients' central nervous system explains at least a part of their better clinical results.

11. INDICATIONS AND TIMING OF SECONDARY REPAIRS

R. Tubiana

The timing of secondary repairs after nerves lesions often presents many problems.

Usually we wait too long before performing secondary repairs. As a result, trophic changes and trick movements have already developed and may be very difficult to correct.

I shall discuss briefly: the signs of nerve regeneration; the prognosis of the various lesions; the indications for secondary repair for motor function and, finally, a few considerations about secondary repair for sensation.

THE SIGNS OF RECOVERY OF NERVE FUNCTION

Recovery proceeds in a proximal to distal direction, sensation recovers before voluntary motor function and the first clinical indication of recovery is Tinel's sign.

The sign is best elicited using a light plessor starting at the level of the nerve suture and proceeding distally. The sign is positive when a patient feels a tingling sensation in the area of skin normally supplied by the nerve. False positives may be prevented by firm digital pressure between the level of percussion and the level of the nerve suture. The value of Tinel's sign is limited as many of the finer fibres reacting in this sign will not reach full recovery.

Theoretically, the axon grows at the rate of 1 mm per day (1 inch per month). In practice, the rate of growth is variable and usually slower. Motor recovery, as previously stated, is always slower than sensory recovery. The first sign is reduction of the muscle atrophy. Next a flicker of activity is detectable which is not powerful enough to overcome gravity. These signs are not in all cases followed by functional recovery.

Skilled *electromyography* will show signs of motor recovery before the appearance of clinical signs of motor recovery; however, Tinel's sign is usually positive before there are signs on the E.M.G. Early electromyographic manifestation, like Tinel's sign, is not a definite sign of 'useful recovery' or that useful recovery will come later.

Whilst it is important to detect the signs of regeneration,

it is much more important to follow the *progress of regeneration*. There are frequent discrepancies between the rate of motor and the rate of sensory recovery. It is important to observe the time interval between visible signs in the muscle nearest the suture line and the next distal muscle. The regeneration may slow down and ultimately stop before it reaches the extremity. All these variants make the assessment of the indication for secondary intervention and the timing of this intervention very difficult.

ASSESSING THE PROGNOSIS

In traumatic lesion, the prognosis depends mainly on the age of the patient, on the delay before active treatment and on the type of lesion.

(a) All statistics show that better results are achieved in children than in adults. The reason for this is not clear but it seems to depend more on the greater adaptability of the child than on an increased potential of nerve regeneration. (E. Almquist, E. A. Orvar).

(b) Statistics show but less conclusively that delay impairs the quality of recovery.

For the motor function, the usual limit for useful recovery appears to be one year after the lesion: for recovery of protective sensation a much longer delay is allowable. In my experience, recovery of protective sensation is possible even after 4 or 5 years. The term protective sensation must not be confused with gnosis which is always difficult to obtain even after early repair.

(c) Local conditions.

In a traumatic lesion, the prognosis will also depend on the site of injury, the loss of nerve substance, associated lesions and the quality of surgery available.

1. *Site*

The more proximal the lesion, the worse the prognosis.

2. *Loss of Nerve Substance*

A significant loss of nerve substance means more difficulties for recovery.

3. *Associated Injuries* of muscle, bone and blood vessels, all lead to scar tissue formation which forms a barrier to effective regeneration.

The treatment is aimed at minimizing the formation of scar tissue, especially by avoiding traction at the level of the repair. Millesi has shown the importance of avoiding traction by the use of fascicular nerve grafts.

Overall, the quality of the treatment is obviously of the greatest importance.

INDICATIONS FOR SECONDARY OPERATIONS

One has to consider, on one hand the possibility of further spontaneous recovery, and on the other the disability caused by the nerve involved.

THE POSSIBILITY OF FURTHER RECOVERY

1. *No Chance of Recovery* (the lesion is too proximal in an adult or because the local conditions are very poor). Even if there is no or negligible possibility of motor recovery, nerve repair can be indicated to achieve protective sensibility.

In cases where secondary treatment should be started as soon as possible, such treatment should be definitive. After a traumatic lesion, it is of course necessary to wait for the inflammatory reaction to subside. In any case, tendon transfers should not be made until scar tissue impeding their gliding function has been replaced and a satisfactory range of passive motion has been obtained. During this period of waiting, the hand must be properly splinted to improve available muscle function and to prevent fixed deformity.

2. *Slight Chance of Recovery.* Recovery will only be functionally poor because of either delayed repair of the nerves or poor conditions for the repair. In these cases the secondary procedure must not be such that it creates its own disability, nor must it jeopardize future function from further nerve recovery.

For example if there is still a slight possibility of recovery, one would not use an important muscle as a transfer, like sublimis but use a less important muscle or another procedure such as a tenodesis or a capsuloplasty.

As an example: after an open fracture of the humerus with laceration of the radial nerve and poor repair, an early transfer of the pronator teres into the wrist extensors was performed because the patient was a pianist; the radial nerve unexpectedly recovered. The patient then developed a hyperextension deformity of the wrist and I had to divide the transfer.

3. *Good Chance of Recovery.* Most surgeons would not consider the possibility of operative intervention, until sufficient time has elapsed to demonstrate failure. However, some surgeons use secondary procedures as 'internal splints' to avoid secondary contractures and cumbersome external splints.

WHAT DISABILITIES CAN BE IMPROVED?

Median Nerve Lesion. Statistics from Zachary, Seddon and Önne show that there is recovery of useful opposition in only about 20–25 per cent of median nerve repairs near the elbow. However good our technique is or may become we are unlikely to improve very much upon this figure, whenever there is significant loss of nerve substance. This is on account of the anatomical complexity of the median nerve.

Delay before secondary intervention. Various authors have suggested different waiting times before secondary intervention. Lange waited 2 years; on the other hand Deyerle and Tucker suggest performing tendon transfers at the same time as the nerve repair. White waits 3–4 months after nerve repair.

I consider it reasonable to wait for about 4 months.

1. *If there is not any sign of recovery*, I would suggest re-exploring the nerve.

If the nerve repair seems of good quality, even after an interfascicular neurolysis, I would wait 2 or 3 more months before doing tendon transfers.

If the repair was poor, I would attempt a new repair, usually a graft at this stage. A tenodesis or some tendon transfer might be considered simultaneously or in the following weeks in adults, if the site of the repair is proximal. In children, I would wait 2 more months.

2. *If 4 months* after the primary nerve repair, there are signs of recovery of sensation, I would wait longer, the precise time depends upon how proximal the site of the lesion is. If *after 6 months* and repeated E.M.G. studies there are no sign of any motor recovery, exploration of the nerve is again indicated.

3. If there is proximal motor recovery but opposition is not recovered, it is inadvisable to wait longer than 9 months and it would probably be advisable to wait less.

It goes without saying that whilst waiting, one must actively prevent the formation of joint stiffness and contractures by physical therapy and splintage. It is of particular importance that the patient should not be allowed to develop the use of the thumb in external rotation and supination. A small lively splint will keep the thumb in the opposed position until the surgeon is ready to decide about an operation. Technically, I would suggest to re-establish only the anteposition of the thumb by the transfer of the extensor pollicis brevis, or even of the palmaris longus prolonged by the palmar aponeurosis.

Ulnar Nerve Lesion. After a proximal ulnar nerve repair the recovery of the intrinsic muscles is often poor. It is often advisable to consider palliative procedures quite early, because,

(a) it is difficult to get useful recovery of intrinsic muscle function following ulnar nerve repair, mainly on account of the distal situation of these muscles.

(b) the metacarpophalangeal joints stiffen rapidly with disuse, especially if they are in hyperextension.

Combined Median and Ulnar Paralyses. The arguments already stated apply with more emphasis here. When there is *no* chance of recovery, the technique of definitive repair to choose shall be discussed later.

When there is a possibility of further recovery, we insist

again that it is important to avoid procedures which will leave irreversible situations, such as arthrodesis or the transfer of important muscles. Early intervention is important as it prevents the development of trick movements which are extremely difficult to correct after late secondary procedures. The two main trick movements to prevent are:

1. The use of the long extensor of the thumb as an adductor, the contraction of which is antagonistic to the action of the muscles of opposition.
2. The habit of flexing the wrist to aid extension of the fingers. I would suggest in paralysis of the thumb, the transfer of an extensor proprius for opposition, using the ulna after excision of the deep fascia as a pulley.

To avoid hyperextension of the metacarpophalangeal joints, I would propose a simple tenodesis, using a graft from the flexor retinaculum to the extensor expansion in the manner described by Athol Parkes. An early anterior capsulorrhaphy of the metacarpophalangeal joint as advocated by Zancolli may sometimes be considered when there are multiple nerves involved, since it does not require a tendon transfer.

Radial Nerve Lesion. For the radial nerve, one has to be even more careful in assessing the indications for early intervention, because recovery is more frequent. This is mainly on account of the proximal situation of the muscles supplied by the radial nerve. In division of the radial nerve at the midhumerus, transfer should be delayed 6 months or longer after neurorraphy. However, while waiting for a possible recovery, it is most important to avoid stiffness of the metacarpophalangeal joints, since this is a serious complication of this paralysis.

SENSORY RECOVERY

Experience has shown that even after late repair of a nerve, useful protective sensation may be recovered. This restricts considerably the use of palliative procedures for recovery of sensation. However, although this protective sensation is very useful, it is not sufficient for special activities in special regions; for instance, a skilled man doing fine work. On the other hand, procedures for the restoration of sensation, such as heterodigital neurovascular island flap transfers, even when technically brilliant, are often far from perfect in their functional results. Ischaemic complications are rare if the operative technique is carefully performed. In 52 personal cases, there was only one distal partial necrosis of the flap and that was traceable to a congenital anomaly of the vascular supply.

On the contrary, troubles in the field of sensibility are frequent and limit considerably the functional value of this procedure. They may be due to compression of the neurovascular bundle or to excessive tension on the flap.

Paraesthesia and pain are not uncommon. The sensitivity of the flap is usually such that two-point discrimination is only slightly reduced. However, if the finger, which has received the flap is not used, through pain, stiffness or unsuitable mental attitude of the patient, the sensation of the flap will not be integrated to its new site and the two-point discrimination will regress. The donor finger is not uninjured in that it has lost half its sensitivity, sometimes presents some pain and contraction may occur in the scar especially when a large flap has been taken. Although we must not minimize these possible complications, we should not let them prevent us from using this procedure which is in some cases the only possible useful operation. In cases where one needs to bring at the same time skin, nutrition and sensation, such as in reconstruction of the thumb, this operation is without equal and usually gives good results. On the other hand, when one only wishes to transfer sensation the indications for this procedure must be severely restricted and carefully assessed for each individual case. In our opinion, this operation is only definitely indicated when a digit with good sensation requires amputation and the skin from this digit can be transferred to an anaesthetic area, or in patients with associated eye damage.

We would also consider sensory transfer in the dominant hand of young, active, intelligent, mentally stable patients who have a median nerve lesion, with good ulnar nerve sensation and a useful pain-free hand, should their occupation require it.

12. NERVE SUTURE TODAY

J. Michon

Repair of the peripheral nerves is still one of the main concerns of any surgeon dealing with reparative surgery of the motor system.

This interest is stimulated by the unknown aspects of the biological problem of nerve regeneration, by technical difficulties which are far from solved, and by the irritating imperfections which still spoil too many of the functional results despite the care taken at the operations and their follow-up.

The author's own modest contribution to this immense subject will be limited to a review of operative technique as it has been modified in concept or execution since the end of the Second World War.

The tendency among most specialists is to achieve precision without injury in carrying out the anastomosis, which today is no longer considered as the mere joining of two elements—the two ends of the nerve trunk—but as the repair of a complex cable, whose multiple elements should ideally be reconnected one by one. Since this microscopic ideal is completely unattainable, technique at the present stage is designed to join one by one the secondary groups of fibres or bundles between the nerve ends. This is already considerably reducing errors in the direction taken by regenerating axons.

Apart from this fundamental problem, many questions arise at all stages in the operation and the author will try to provide an answer to them, although fully aware that in many respects we are still at the stage of only tentative conclusions.

SURGICAL EXPLORATION AT THE TIME OF THE INJURY

(A) EMERGENCY CASES

There is scarcely any need to recall here that any wound crossed by a nerve trunk requires investigation and exploration of the nerve to the same extent as when we are dealing with a vascular pedicule, a joint or a tendon.

As we shall see, even though primary suture is not necessarily always to be recommended, at least the damage to the nerve must be seen and dressed and the two nerve ends brought together by means of two easily identified sutures so as to avoid retraction. All this must be strictly noted in the operation report.

(B) SECONDARY SURGERY

In the case of a secondary operation in a scar area, exploration of the one or more nerve trunks must proceed from the simple to the complex: uncovering the nerves above and below the lesions and a gradual dissection towards the scar area.

The appearance of the nerve lesion is often unambiguous when there is a separation of the two cut ends or when, on the other hand, the nerve trunk is intact but is simply compressed in a scar or by a fracture callus.

In a certain number of cases, however, examination of the lesion itself does not resolve the problem of diagnosis. So-called lesions 'in continuity' may correspond to different degrees of damage with a different prognosis, depending on whether or not there exists a real continuity of the nerve sheaths and axons inside the scar (Fig. 12.1). The diagram very roughly shows what can be concealed in an indurated olive-shaped swelling or in a lateral nodule. It is quite obvious that a dense internal scar justifies complete or partial redissection of the nerve followed by suture, whereas an intraneural or perineural scar fibroma only requires an excision which preserves the continuity of the nerve bundles, using intraneural dissection.

Some neurophysiological investigations during operations are now being studied: direct measurement of nerve conduction by means of electrodes applied directly to the nerve trunk above and below the lesion may perhaps one day provide valuable information on the continuity of the differentiated elements of the nerve. In the same way measurement during the operation of the rate of conduction of the nerve impulse is a valid quantitative test of the continuity of the axons. The practical technique of these studies and the apparatus used require further development and improvement, but soon such methods will be part of current practice. It should be noted that the results of the measurements are only reliable for a short time after inflation of the pneumatic tourniquet.

Intraneural dissection often remains the only method of diagnosing the lesion which will determine the prognosis

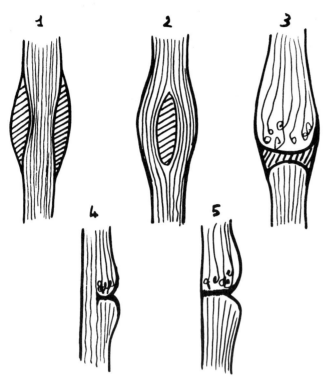

Figure 12.1
Nerve lesions with apparent continuity: in an olive-shaped swelling may or may not the continuity of the fibres be preserved and a lateral notch corresponds to partial or total section of the nerve trunk.

and the steps to be taken. The dissection can be carried out longitudinally along the axis of the trunk, the bundles being freed from the adherent scar above and below and also inside the nodule itself. This technique has the disadvantage of splitting up the healthy nerve ends and making suture difficult if this should be necessary after the investigation. Where there is a gap in nerve continuity the bundles inside the scar are lost in a mesh of fine branches. According to Seddon, transverse intraneural dissection is to be preferred. While the nerve scar is kept under tension a sharp blade is used to cut transversely and remove piece by piece the hard resistant scar tissue. When healthy nerve tissue is reached, it pouches out since it is suddenly freed from the constraint of the scar. These healthy zones should then be left intact and freed from the area of operation. With patience it is possible to find the healthy bundles in a partial wound, to free a nerve trunk under compression or, on the other hand, to demonstrate the presence of a complete anatomical gap in the nerve trunk. Action can then be taken which is fully adapted to the lesions.

From this stage of the operation onwards, the use of magnifying apparatus makes it possible to get a much more precise picture of the nerve tissue and its lesions. The author has performed neurolysis of the digital nerves in

scar where the naked eye would not have been able to detect and isolate these nerves, although they were intact.

Upon concluding this exploratory stage in the operation in a certain number of cases treatment is practically completed: the nerve is freed from external compression and from its own scars. There is nothing left to do but to leave it in a bed of healthy tissue with good vascularization: connective tissue, fat or muscle.

In other patients, however, there are indications that nerve repair by suture or graft is required.

CURRENT CONCEPTS OF NERVE SUTURE

In a histological cross-section of a nerve, it is striking to note the importance of the connective tissue spaces in relation to the bundles of nerve fibres.

The epineurium only appears as a special appendage of the neighbouring connective tissue with which it is continuous, and not as the distinct sheath which it is usually imagined to be. On the other hand, every intraneural bundle possesses its own sheath or perineurium which seems denser and more autonomous than the epineurium.

According to Sunderland's ideas, every bundle is a sort of preview of a collateral or terminal branch of the trunk but exchanges of fibres between the bundles are numerous and occur at many levels and the bundles cross each other in such a way that a systematic picture of their respective positions is very difficult to obtain as a guide for surgery.

As surgeons, we know however that it is possible to continue dissection and separation of a nerve branch inside a trunk for 10 or 15 cm.

In practice the problem with which we are faced is how to bring the two sections of a nerve face to face so that the regeneration of the axons can be properly oriented.

It is important that as many as possible of the efferent fibres which are to terminate in muscles should be directed to the appropriate sheaths and that the afferent sensory fibres should end in the correct peripheral receptors.

The best way of avoiding errors of direction seems to be to substitute for the concept of the trunk suture that of the fascicular suture with the aim of bringing face to face the same bundles in the two halves of the nerve.

Sunderland, who was the first to advocate this concept of nerve suture, is still however, pessimistic regarding the practical possibilities of carrying it out.

In fact the difficulty varies according to situation: the nearer the lesion to the root of the limb, the more numerous the bundles and the more anarchical their arrangement, so that finding them is difficult and uncertain. On the other hand, distally the number of fascicles is reduced and their arrangement is more regular and constant, so that it becomes easier to find them and orientation can be more confident. Thus, in the lower third of the forearm the structure of the ulnar nerve is quite clearly visible, with three or four bundles which can be identified on the basis of their differences in diameter.

TECHNIQUE FOR FASCICULAR SUTURE

(A) APPARATUS

Since 1961, the author has achieved greater technical precision by the use of magnifying spectacles, but in 1964, during a stay in the U.S.A., he visited J. W. Smith, an assistant of Conway, who was repairing the nerves and tendons of the hand under a dissecting microscope, and became convinced that this was correct.

Since that time the microscope has formed an essential part of the author's surgical equipment. He believes that its use is irreplaceable not only to discover the best possible orientation for the bundles, but also to evaluate the thickness of the epineurium and the degree of precision of the

approximation of the ends and the tension of the sutures.

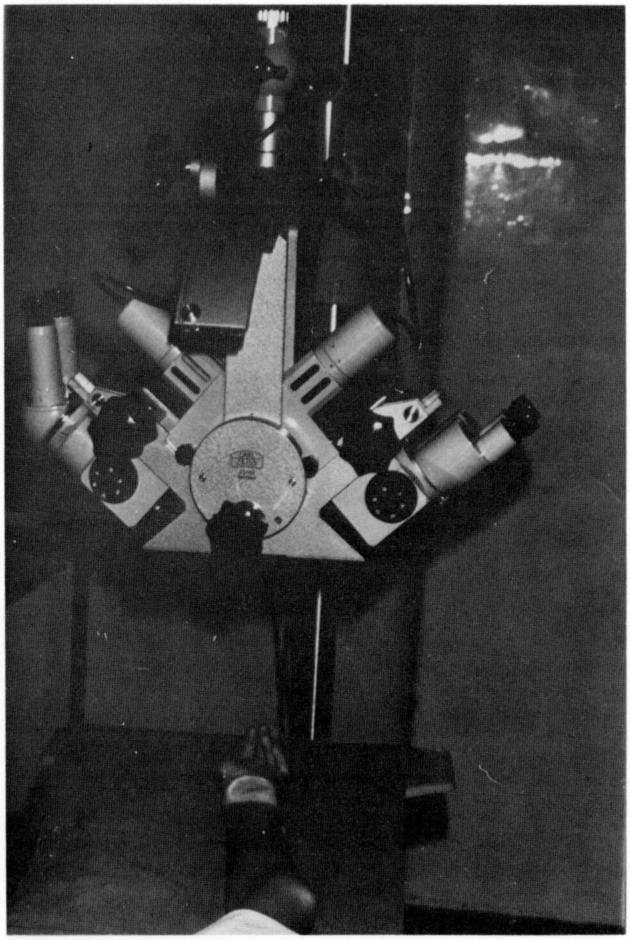

We have at the moment two types of optical equipment available: a table-model binocular loupe in which changing of the lenses provides different magnifications (this apparatus, together with its stand, can be sterilized with formalin or ethylene oxide) and a dissecting microscope with two viewing positions (diploscope, Fig. 12.2), the magnification it provides being varied by moving a threaded sleeve. Mounted on a stand with wheels, this apparatus is excellent for teaching this type of surgery but, apart from the controls, cannot be sterilized.

(B) PREPARATION OF NERVE ENDS

If the nerve lesion or scar is considered beyond repair, it is essential to obtain at each end a section exactly perpendicular to the axis and completely flat and regular.

The quality of the apposition depends on this recutting. Some very important research by Edshage has shown in experimental sections the frequency of poor apposition with massive losses of axons which are twisted and put out of line and never reach the nerve sheaths of the distal portion again if the recutting has been badly done.

Since then a certain number of ingenious pieces of

Figure 12.2
A diploscope making it possible for the surgeon and his assistant to observe the procedure.

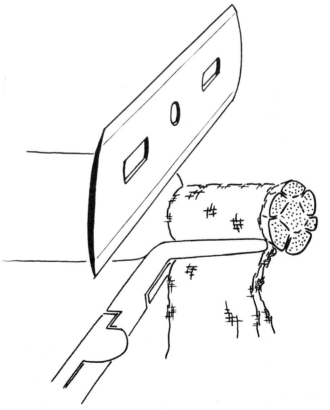

Figure 12.3
Resection of a nerve ending by the Jean Gosset technique.

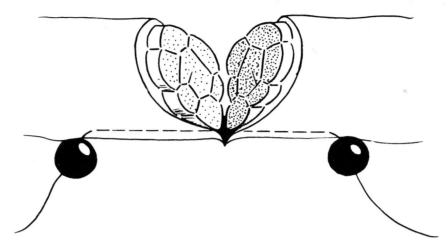

Figure 12.4 Immobilization of the nerve ends by means of a thread and two sinkers (J. Gosset).

apparatus have been developed to immobilize the nerve and enable it to be cut by guillotine. The author personally uses the method of Jean Gosset, who ensheathes the nerve in a ribbon of elastic plastic clamped by means of a biangular forceps so that it is ready for cutting with a blade (Fig. 12.3). The surface obtained in this way is clean and not bruised and there is no interference with the fascicular structure.

Work under high magnification requires that the segments to be joined should be completely immobilized and here again the ingenuity of Jean Gosset has provided us with a useful technique: a thread passed through the epineurium of the two portions of nerve is blocked with two heavy angler's sinkers. It brings the two ends together and immobilizes them in the microscope field (Fig. 12.4).

(C) THE FASCICULAR SUTURE

To enable the fascicular pattern of the two nerve ends to be seen clearly, impregnation with a solution of dilute methylene blue appreciably improves the contrast. The main bundles are distinguished in each half by means of their different diameters and 'geographical' position.

Interfascicular sutures are then inserted atraumatically through the epineurium and penetrate deeply into the connective tissue septa. These sutures will guide apposition and prevent axial rotation (Fig. 12.5).

Some think that the same orientation can be obtained by simply inserting epineural stitches (Fig. 12.6). We consider that the great mobility of the bundles inside the epineurium makes this method less precise.

Other surgeons, such as Millesi, place the suture threads on the fascicular sheaths themselves (the perineurium) (Fig. 12.7). The author, however, prefers to avoid leaving knots, however small, inside the nerve trunk.

When all the sutures needed to make the direction of the bundles precise have been inserted, they are tied under only moderate tension. Suture is then completed with sutures on the epineurium, the whole operation being carried out under

the microscope, with the utmost possible care, gentleness and precision.

The author uses single threads of nylon of 8 or 10/0 fitted in swaged ophthalmic needles. This material looked at under a magnification of 12 or 24 still seems much too thick and a great deal of progress remains to be made in this respect.

INDICATIONS FOR OPERATION

It is first of all necessary to take up a position on the fiercely disputed point regarding the best time for nerve repair. Everyone knows that the more time that elapses, the worse are the chances of effective regeneration because of the occlusion of the empty nerve sheaths and above all the atrophy of the muscles, even if the sensory receptors seem to be endowed with a capacity for extremely long survival. However, these degenerative phenomena take place late enough for it to be possible to hesitate between primary repair, when the cutaneous wound is closed, and secondary repair, between 3 weeks and 3 months after the injury, a lapse of time indicated by Seddon and most of the Anglo-Saxon authors and defended in France by Merle d'Aubigné.

However, it must be recognized that Jean Gosset is right in saying that a number of primary sutures gave good results.

The biological arguments put forward in the 1954 report of the British Medical Research Council hardly stand up to the criticisms of modern neurophysiologists although the technical arguments are much more sound. Scar formation thickens the perineural and intraneural laminae of connective tissue, making it easier to determine the fascicular structure and conferring more stability on the suture.

Above all, however, secondary surgery can be carried out in infinitely better conditions than emergency surgery and with less risk of infection.

A priori, in contused wounds where the vitality of the

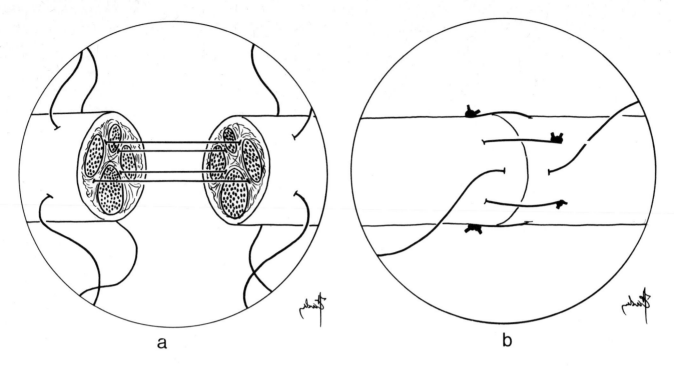

Figure 12.5
Orientation by means of interfascicular sutures:
(a) insertion of interfascicular stitches;
(b) terminal epineural suture.

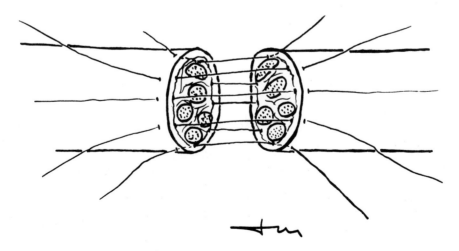

Figure 12.6
Orientation of the bundles by means of simple epineural suture.
In the author's opinion this lacks precision.

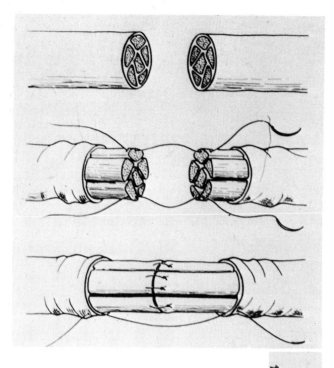

Figure 12.7
Fascicular perineural suture (Millesi).

tissues is in doubt and the risk of sepsis is high, no emergency nerve repair can be recommended. The point of view here is the same as, or perhaps even more strict than, in the case of sutures of flexor tendons.

On the other hand, in clean incised wounds in the hand for example, primary repair of the pure sensory terminal branches or pure muscular terminal branches gives sufficiently consistent results to make it unreasonable to put off the operation in order to make the technical side of it easier.

It is in the case of the mixed nerve trunks that the question has not yet been settled and both points of view have fervent supporters. The author's own point of view is cautious and flexible and he considers the indications for primary suture to be restricted and precise:

1. Accidental section of a nerve trunk during a surgical operation.
2. Section of nerves in attempted suicide where psychological conditions are unfavourable for secondary surgery.
3. Partial, incomplete lesions of the nerve trunks where secondary resection can be a very delicate operation and late repair can be difficult.

In all other cases the author prefers to carry out secondary repair as soon as the conditions of the scar provide sufficient security from infection and from trophic risks.

The choice between nerve suture and nerve grafts obviously depends on the question of the apparent or actual loss of substance. Injury, ischaemia and sclerosis, the retraction of the nerve ending and surgical resection are the usual causes.

Suture leads to a longitudinal tension which, if it is excessive, may entail failure or sclerosis of the anastomosis (Millesi).

This tension can be reduced by extensive dissection of the nerve with freeing of the collateral branches inside the trunk but the risk of ischaemia makes it essential not to run too far in this direction. It is possible to eliminate temporarily any traction on the suture by putting the neighbouring joints in flexion during the 3 weeks necessary for scar formation, but the secondary elongation which will then occur is not without its disadvantages and in the author's practice has had a very damaging influence in certain cases (see the thesis of P. Masse, Nancy, 1961).

Some surgeons, like Millesi, end by recommending nerve grafts in almost every case, and while the author refuses to follow them in such an extreme point of view he believes that the indications for grafts should be extended and that in sutures only a moderate tension should be accepted compatible with physiological joint posture: 50° at the elbow, 30° at the wrist and 70° at the knee (Fig. 12.8).

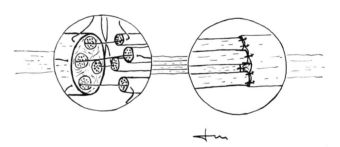

Figure 12.8
Fascicular grafts under the microscope.

CONCLUSIONS

The author cannot at the moment provide statistical results affording definite proof that his techniques are sound and it will take several years before such long-term results can be provided.

He hopes that this paper will leave the reader with the conviction that we must be very demanding in regard to ourselves and the results we obtain. Our aim must not be to obtain beautiful photographic slides for meetings of learned societies, but really functional results which make our patients normal workers whose hands in their work and their daily life will fulfil their role of providing sensory information and acting as an automatic tool. This ideal is less often attained than many think or are willing to admit.

13. EXPOSURE OF NERVES IN THE UPPER LIMB

F. Iselin

For nerve repair work, the surgical exposure must be carefully designed in relation to the presumed site of the lesion and existing scars.

It must be possible to enlarge them, if need be, in a way determined beforehand so that the damaged nerve can always be found on either side of the lesion, since dissection must always move from the known towards the unknown, from the distant normal portions towards the area of scarring or the lesion.

Whether it is an old or a new lesion that is being repaired, the general pattern of incision is identical, for even with a fresh wound its debridement, which is essential, should be brought in line as far as possible with the ideal pathway of approach to the nerve or nerves to be repaired.

Most of the mistakes and accidents that occur are the result of operations carried out along approaches which are inadequate or badly placed.

APPROACH TO THE AXILLARY NERVES

Since lesions of the brachial plexus are in most cases irreparable, we shall restrict ourselves to describing an approach which enable high repair of the three nerves at their origin in the lower part of the armpit.

The patient should be in the dorsal decubitus position on the operating table with his arm abducted at 90° and with a cushion under his shoulder.

The cutaneous incision runs parallel to the lower border of the pectoralis major along its whole course, a distance of 10–12 cm from the apex of the axilla.

The thin axillary fascia will be found and opened, allowing the lower border of the pectoralis major to be retracted and the sheath of the coraco-brachialis to be exposed. An incision is made in the posterior border of the muscle, which is also retracted.

The neurovascular bundle is situated immediately below and is easily accessible.

THE ARM

APPROACH TO THE RADIAL NERVE

To reach the radial trunk the posterior median approach is the best, particularly because it can be carried further down and outwards towards the lateral cubital fossa.

The patient should be lying supine, with the arm abducted at 90° and resting on a cradle with the forearm hanging down allowing its rotation by an assistant.

A posterior median incision is made from the lower border of the deltoid to three-fingers' breadth above the olecranon.

Once an incision has been made in the muscular aponeurosis, the radial groove is exposed from the top of the incision and displayed from top to bottom by separating the two muscle bellies.

APPROACH TO THE MEDIAN AND ULNAR NERVES

Here it is sufficient to make a skin incision along the medial border of the biceps to the medial epicondyle to have an excellent view of the median nerve. Incision of the medial intermuscular aponeurosis readily exposes the ulnar nerve behind it.

THE ELBOW

THE MEDIAN NERVE

The median nerve is exposed by making a medial bicipital approach along the border of the biceps tendon. An incision parallel to the border and extending to the upper third of the forearm uncovers the median basilic vein, which is retracted. The bicipital aponeurosis crosses the incision obliquely. It is sectioned from top to bottom starting from its upper border, which is easily found at the top of the incision. The nerve bundle is just below and the median nerve lies medially as it passes downwards into the pronator teres under the flexor digitorum sublimis muscle.

THE ULNAR NERVE

The ulnar nerve is in the epitrochleo-olecranon sulcus which is approached through a vertical incision made equidistant from the two bony prominences. An incision is made in the muscle sheath and the nerve is just below, against the medial epicondyle. It passes under the flexor carpi ulnaris muscle in the lower part. It is this muscle whose upper insertion must be incised so that the nerve can be transposed in front of the medial epicondyle. The insertion is then reconstituted behind the transposed nerve.

THE RADIAL NERVE

This is in the lateral cubital fossa. The incision is made along the lateral edge of the biceps tendon to expose the median cephalic vein. The musculocutaneous nerve emerges on the external margin of the biceps and must be retracted within the incision.

The radial nerve is at the bottom of the gap between the brachioradialis muscle on the outside and the brachialis muscle on the inside, about 1 cm outside the biceps tendon.

The superficial branch follows the brachioradialis muscle in its sheath, while the motor branch, the ramus profundus, makes its way between the two heads of the supinator muscle at a distance of 1 cm below the cubital fossa.

THE FOREARM

Here we are dealing only with lesions of the median and ulnar nerve trunks.

THE MEDIAN NERVE

The skin incision continues in the direction of the medial bicipital groove, crosses the axis of the forearm in its upper third and goes on vertically or slightly obliquely towards the outer border.

The nerve is just under the muscle sheath and makes its way through the pronator teres, which must be retracted firmly medially and relaxed by placing the limb in maximum pronation. Lower down the nerve to flexor digitorum superficialis, along the deep edge of which it makes its way, must be retracted. Further down still, the incision will continue to the inner border of the tendon of the flexor carpi radialis muscle, just behind which lies the nerve.

THE ULNAR NERVE

This is exposed by means of a curved skin incision moving from one side to the other of a baseline which runs from the apex of the medial epicondyle to the outer border of the pisiform bone. During the whole length of its course the nerve is deep to the flexor carpi ulnaris, along the inner border of the flexor digitorum sublimis muscle. Below, of course, there are two aponeuroses to go through at the anterior border of the flexor carpi ulnaris muscle before the nerve bundle can be found.

WRIST AND HAND

Here the ending of the two nerves is approached through a bayonet incision which; if adequate exposure is carried out, allows complete inspection of the various elements without leaving contracted scars across the flexion creases (Fig. 13.1)

Generally speaking, the incision will be transverse in one of the flexion creases of the hand, longitudinal along the opposition crease of the thumb, and a transverse one in the flexion crease of the wrist or oblique longitudinal one in the forearm. The angles will be rounded as much as possible to

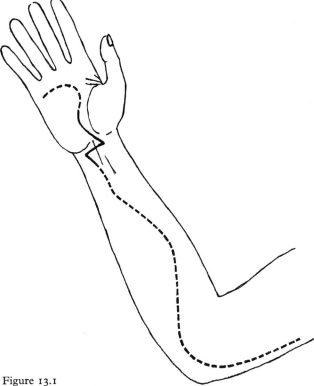

Figure 13.1

avoid sloughing. The flaps will be given minimum dissection and their subcutaneous fatty layer must be conserved. The nerves are very near the surface in the palm and are the first elements encountered after the subcutaneous fat. In the wrist the median nerve is situated below the flexor retinaculum, which will have to be opened over a cannula inserted in the carpal tunnel.

THE FINGERS

We have abandoned the classical incision along the mid–lateral line, since this pathway follows the very course of the digital nerve, which may be involved in the resultant scar. Furthermore, we have seen several cases of volar contracture.

We have therefore moved the incision back towards the dorsal surface at its line of junction with the lateral surface. It is thus a dorsolateral incision (Figs. 13.2, 13.3).

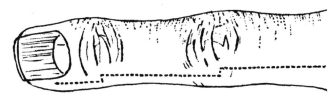

Figure 13.2

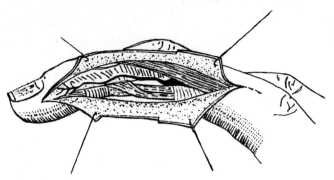

Figure 13.3

To facilitate healing of this incision we stagger it slightly from phalanx to phalanx, so that while frankly dorsal at P1 it has become almost lateral at P3 (Fig. 13.3). Combined if need be with a transverse palmar incision, this approach gives excellent exposure of the tendons and of *both* digital nerves. This is done at the expense of considerable detachment of tissue, but this is no disdavantage.

14. RECENT ADVANCES IN THE FIELD OF MICROSURGERY

James W. Smith

Recent reports, both experimental and clinical (Ito, Goto, Hirotani, Tamura, Buncke, Grabb, Hakstian) confirm the fact that repairing peripheral nerves under magnification is increasing both the speed of returning nerve function and its quality. A second area of major advancement is appearing in the field of instrumentation. As the smaller instruments of the ophthalmologist and otolaryngologist were found more helpful than the standard one of general surgical size, we now see such microminiature equipment as metallized microsutures, electronically controlled microsurgical instruments, and a triploscope. This latter instrument makes it possible for two assistants to share the same optical advantages as the operator (O'Brien). A single foot control adjusts the focus and magnification.

More portable microscopes are also being developed for procedures requiring magnification for the operator. Such instruments as the Mentor CM-11 have the advantages of simplicity and ease of operation, low cost and portability. This microscope can be removed from its small carrying case and quickly attached by a clamp to the operating table. Magnifications of $10\times$, $-15\times$, and $20\times$ are possible, simply by changing the oculars.

Another lightweight microscope is held on the head with an adjustable head band. It can be raised out of the way by an assistant when magnification is not needed.

A third major advancement has been made in the field with the advent of fascicular suturing. Proposed by Sunderland and described by Goto, it appears to give results superior to those achieved by simple epineural repair.

It is unfortunate that we have no way to tell how successfully the regeneration process is proceeding a month or two after the operation. Then if we could project the future result, it would not only benefit the patient, but also would aid greatly in assessing results without having to wait so long. At present, only after a period of from 3 to 5 years can an accurate estimate of the success of the surgery be established, for it takes that long to regain the maximum of muscle function and sensation almost regardless of the level of the injury.

Perhaps we should feel fortunate that we can get *any* return of function or sensation because, of all the nerves of the body, only those in the peripheral system have the power of regeneration.

Yet, we need to know more about the true capacity of this system to regenerate—what percentage of its normal functioning state we can expect will be lost from injury on the basis of limited regenerative powers and what percentage on the basis of technical inadequacy at the time of repair.

In other words is regeneration limited by the inability of some nerve cells to attain a sufficiently high level of proteosynthesis to completely repair the damaged axon and restore it to its original state? Or, is the potential for total axonal regeneration actually present, but never achieved because of such mechanical factors as scarring, fascicular kinking and slight malalignment. The fact that Ito *et al.* have found levels of return approaching normal in some of their cases is strong evidence in favour of there being a potential for great amounts of regeneration—if more of the mechanical factors can be solved. The cell body for each of those motor end plates out in the extremity is located within the spinal cord. The cell body for sensory nerves is located in the posterior root ganglion. From these rather central sites, axons extend out into the extremities over lengths of up to 3 feet. This is an extremely long distance when one considers that nerve cells have a body size of 20–100 μm and an axonal cross section of 8–20 μm. Against the argument that the length of these nerve communication lines and their regenerative capacities represents the total answer, is the fact that a complete recovery can be expected with certain types of nerve injury, regardless of the level at which they occur. An example is found in neuropraxia (Seddon, 1943) where there is an interruption of axonal condution, usually caused by pressure, but with preservation of anatomical continuity. While the loss of sensory and motor function may last for a few days or even several months time, the recovery will be complete.

The same is true of axonotmesis (Seddon, 1943), the type of crush injury in which there is a loss of continuity of the axons but no disruption of the endoneurium. Although Wallerian degeneration of the axons occurs distal to the point of the injury, the endoneural tubes are preserved, so that when axons begin to regenerate after a few days, they are directed back down through their tubes to the end organ they originally ennervated.

However, when the injury results in the disruption in both the fasciculus and its surrounding perineurium, the chances of a good recovery decrease markedly. Even though the epineurium remains intact, thereby maintaining the physical continuity of the nerve, the regenerating axons often enter the wrong endoneural tubes or even grow into the interfascicular spaces where they will end blindly. Regeneration is so severely compromised under the circumstances that a spontaneous recovery to a useful level in these cases is rare. An excision of the involved segment and a suture repair is usually required.

Since most injuries less severe than this usually have a good prognosis, while the ones which are more severe have an extremely bad prognosis, it would seem that the perineurium somehow plays a major role in the problem of regeneration.

ANATOMY

Each peripheral nerve contains a great number of nerve fibres or axons, individually enclosed within an endoneurial sheath. These units are in turn bound together into bundles or fascicules by adjacent connective tissue, the perineurium. Surrounding a group of the bundles is a loose arealar connective tissue framework called the epineurium. The epineurium serves as a definitive external sheath which separates the nerve from surrounding tissues. It contains collagen and elastin fibres, most of which run longitudinally. The endoneurium, perineurium, and epineurium constitute the connective tissue component of a peripheral nerve and each aids in isolating or insulating one part from another. Each also has specific architectural or structural characteristics which deserve consideration.

In his study of the comparative amounts of connective tissue in cross sectional areas of nerves, Sunderland found the smallest amount to be about 22 per cent while the greatest was 88 per cent. In general then, anywhere from 30 to 75 per cent of a peripheral nerve is made up of connective tissue, depending upon the nerve and specific level being examined. There appears to be more connective tissue when the neural components are small and numerous and less when the bundles are few or of a larger size. There is also more at those sites where peripheral nerves pass across joints.

The endoneurium, which surrounds each axon–Schwann cell complex is mostly composed of collagenous tissue. This supporting connective tissue also forms the fine, intra-fascicular septal that separate and subdivide nerve fibres inside a fasciculus into even smaller groups of components. These septa contain the interfascicular blood supply.

The perineurium invests each bundle or fasciculus with a relatively thin but dense and distinctive sheath of fibrous tissue. It contains elastin and collagen fibres which intermesh by passing circularly, obliquely and longitudinally.

The fibrils form from seven to fifteen concentric lamellae or tubes. The number decides the size of the fasciculus or bundle. When one carefully examines the fasciculus in the end of a freshly cut nerve it will be seen that they have the ability to move back and forth independently within the perineurium. The epineurium also has an independence of motion in relation to the other two structures, making the entire unit an unstable composite of about the same quality as well cooked spaghetti. Each piece of spaghetti looks like a fasciculus and has just about as much ability to bend and kink on itself. Injection studies show that between each fasciculus the microcirculation to each runs in the perineurium.

The internal circulation of the nerve arrives through the mesoneurium in a manner similar to that of the intestine. All the nutrient vessels enter the nerve along the line where the mesoneurium attaches to the nerve. No vessels enter the nerve around the remainder of its circumference. Blood is supplied in a segmental fashion, being both dispersed and collected through a series of arcades within the mesoneurium. The grouping of arcades seems to change from one area to another to meet needs and requirements imposed by local anatomical variations. In areas such as the shoulder, elbow, and wrist, where great degrees of mobility are required of the nerve, the mesoneurium is longer, is more complex, and contains more vessels. When there is little or no tension on these vessels, they contract in an accordion-like arrangement. As tension increases with movement, the vessels within the mesoneurium uncoil to accommodate for the changing position of the nerve. The nutrient vessels entering a given portion of nerve through the mesoneurium will, therefore, appear to vary in number depending upon the position of the limb and the degree to which they are stretched. Peripheral nerves possess considerable strength and elasticity. Though it is not possible to isolate and separate the mechanical properties of each component part of a peripheral nerve, much of the tensile strength and elasticity of nerve trunks is derived from the perineurium. It plays a major role in maintaining the integrity of the nerve trunk under tension.

If both the endoneurial and perineurium tube are ruptured by injury the Schwann cells and axons will proliferate in an attempt to repair the damage. Since neither of them is now confined to the tube they will form outgrowths at the point where the tube is severed. According to Denny Brown (see page 85) fibroblasts from the endoneurium and perineurium are solely responsible for the outgrowth of cells at the nerve ends. Thus neuromas can occur even when there is continuity of the nerve, if the endoneurium and perineurium are ruptured.

TIME OF REPAIR

Nearly everyone seems to agree now that in the military type of wound nerve repairs should be performed as a secondary procedure. However, most civilian injuries are caused by glass or sharp knives. Many authors are in favour of primary nerve repairs when these injuries are located in the distal part of an extremity and the trauma is localized (Grabb, 1968; Ducker, Kempe and Hayes, 1969; McEwan, 1962; Sunderland, 1968).

Yet Nicholson and Seddon (1957) and others found in reviewing their series of cases that an early secondary suture offered equally good prospects of recovery as a primary repair. Nicholson states that secondary suturing is more reliable because at that time the epineurium is two to four times its normal thickness and holds sutures well.

A fine experimental study by Grabb (1968) supports those who believe that in civilian wounds, when circumstances permit, the primary repair of a divided nerve yields the best results. Still, most surgeons experienced in this type of work will agree that an inexperienced surgeon will have a far greater chance of getting a poor result after a primary repair than he will after a secondary repair. Why is this so? It is no doubt related, in part, to the fact that the connective tissues in and around the freshly cut nerve are normally quite filmy. Their appearance and future holding power are far less than they would be at the time of a secondary repair. Furthermore, the fasciculi, themselves, are more flexible immediately after a nerve injury. They also can be pulled in and out of the exposed end of the cut nerve with a greater degree of independent mobility than at the time of the secondary repair. Thus, the inexperienced surgeon trying to do a primary repair may more easily shred and fragment the nerve ends into a number of separate fascicules. When an insufficient amount of connective tissue remains between these fascicules, the only thing to do to relieve frustrations and complete the repair is to place sutures right through the fasciculi. If those sutures being used in the repair are not sufficiently small, the prognosis will be jeopardized even more severely, than it was by the injury alone.

These circumstances are quite a contrast to the strong thickened perineurium and epineurium usually found at the time of the second repair. The fascicules seem to be more rigid, to have less independent movement and are more fixed in position in the interface. This tends to diminish their tendency to kink or get angulated at the time of suturing as well as producing a better holding surface for the sutures being used in repair.

METABOLIC CONSIDERATIONS IN NERVE REPAIR

Advocates of a delayed primary repair have appeared in recent years to favour delaying the repair of any injured nerve for at least 4–21 days. There has been great emphasis on the metabolism of nerve cells and their axons in support of the thesis. Some of these points are:

1. When an axon is severed in a peripheral nerve injury, its cell body progressively enlarges for ten to twenty-days, remains enlarged while active regeneration is taking place and then slowly returns to normal size (Ducker, Kempe and Hayes, 1969). This enlargement accompanies an increase in cell metabolism, an increase in enzymic activity, the rate of incorporation of amino acids, the speed at which RNA is transformed into its more active form, and an increased total amount of nucleac acid in the cell bodies (Brattgård, Edström and Hyden, 1958; Edström, 1959; and Gutmann, 1961).

Proteins form in the nerve cell body during this time and begin to migrate down the axon to the site of injury where they aid in regeneration. Experiments show that, in young rats, proteins migrate down axons at a rate of 1·5 millimeters per day and in adult rats at 0·8 millimeters per day (Droz and Leblond, 1963).

2. Injured peripheral nerves heal in two distinct phases: (a) the phase of neuronal survival; and (b) the phase of neuronal regeneration. The phase of neuronal survival can vary from 4 to 20 days. The phase of neuronal regeneration can last from 60 to 300 days, (Drucker, Kempe and Hayes, 1969).

3. There are metabolic changes in the nerve proximal and distal to the point where it has been divided. As both ends of the cut nerve swell, the cross sectional area of each increases three to four times. This swelling extends for about 1 centimetre above and below the point of division and persists for a week or more before subsiding (Drucker and Hayes, 1968).

4. Wallerian degeneration, strictly speaking, is supposed to occur only distal to the site of injury. The axons and the myelin surrounding it, undergo physical disintegration, while the other remaining structures in the peripheral nerve segment (sheath of Schwann, endoneurium, blood vessels, and so forth,) are not destroyed, but remain intact. About one week after the injury macrophages begin to move in and phagocytize the disintegrating axons and myelin. This process extends throughout the distal cut segment and is completed within a 5 to 8 weeks period, ultimately leaving behind the empty and somewhat shrunken sheath of Schwann (Sunderland, 1968; Cajal, 1928). If no repair is done and axons fail to enter the distal segment, its cross sectional area becomes reduced to a point where they are about 1 per cent of normal size at the end of a 2 year period. (Sunderland-Bradley, 1950).

5. The nerve segment just proximal to the point of injury undergoes what Cajal (1928) has termed traumatic degeneration. This is essentially the same as Wallerian degeneration, differing only that it is limited in its extend to just a few millimeters proximal to the point of nerve injury. Axonal budding begins from this site about 4 days after injury when the cut is sharp and the point of injury is located at the more distal parts of the nerve. If the nerve division is quite proximal in the limb and caused by blunt trauma, it may be delayed and may not begin for twenty days. During the time when the axon is regenerating there is vigorous outgrowth of chords of Schwann cells from both the proximal and distal cut ends of the nerve. These cells become surrounded by endoneural and perineural cells to form

numerous small fascicules (Thomas and Jones, 1966, 1967).

When nerves are repaired months or years after injury the cell body and axon undergo the metabolic changes which accompany repair, but the response to the second time is not with the same maximal metabolic effort as the first (Alexsandrovskaya, 1956). Yahr and Beebe (1956) thought after reviewing some patients with nerve injuries during World War II, that nerve repairs performed later than 10 days post injury resulted in a loss of motor return which averaged 1 per cent of maximal function for every 6 days of delay.

Nicholson and Seddon, on the other hand have stated that no apparent harm resulted from a delay of up to 6 months from the time of injury.

In actual clinical experience the early secondary repair seems to be the worst time possible for nerve repair. Circumstances have necesitated, on a number of occasions, that I repair divided nerves 2 to 4 weeks after they were severed. At the time of operation, the nerve was difficult to dissect free from the surrounding indurated connective tissue. The nerve itself was quite firm and it proved to be exceedingly difficult to determine the proximal and distal sites where the nerve was not damaged and would prove suitable for the repair. In cases where the nerve needed to be mobilized to get the ends together, it proved to be quite difficult because of the reaction within the nerve. In several instances the nerve was far more friable than it would have been, had several additional weeks time been allowed between the time of the accident and the time of repair. An additional factor, which seems to argue against delaying nerve repairs in the ideal cases is the fact that the neuroma which forms on the 'nerve ends' actually extends to involve more proximal and distal segments of the nerve. This necessitates a wider resection and the loss of an even greater segment of nerve. So, the two fresh ends which are secondarily approximated are less likely to be similar or have as much matching as between the two original ends.

The epineurial repair of a nerve can appear to be excellent but this gives comparatively little knowledge about the accuracy of fascicular contact within the nerve. If an experimental nerve juncture is frozen and a section taken through it, the external suggestion of accuracy will be replaced by the internal appearance of disaster. The proximal fasciculi are too often poorly aligned with those corresponding on the distal side of the anastomosis. They also can be kinked or misdirected into adjacent epineurium, the insulating material which lies between fasciculi. Since the amount of this insulating material (epineurium) can vary from 20 to 80 per cent of the total cross sectional area of the nerve, the importance of accurate alignment increases as the neural content falls.

The possibility of proximal and distal fasciculi being properly aligned at the time of nerve repair becomes less and less, and the alignment of fasciculi becomes even more of a problem as the number of months increases. The distal component parts become more atrophied and dis-

similar and this of course lessens their chances of matching up with corresponding fasciculi in the proximal segment.

NERVE REPAIR

When a peripheral nerve has been divided, it may be difficult to find the ends in a fresh injury if one only studies the cut surface. They tend to retract back from the wound edge due to the elasticity of the mesoneurium. Perhaps the easiest way to find the ends of a divided nerve, especially at the time of secondary repair, is to look proximal and distal to the point of injury, where the tissues have not been altered by the injury or scar. The surgeon must force himself to begin the dissection in this area and to trace the nerve ends into the area of injury or scar. Once they are located, the cut ends should be tagged with a suture so that they will be easy to recognize.

In cases where the viability of a part is in jeopardy, vascular repair takes precedence over any nerve surgery and the latter should be considered only when it will neither decrease the chance for survival of the part nor appreciably increase the chance for a complication or infection.

In those cases where a nerve repair is to be deferred until a later date, it is important to approximate the nerve ends with a single suture to aid in their later identification and prevent retraction. If a small segment of nerve is missing so that the ends cannot be approximated, the ends should be tacked to the bed or some other fixed structure to keep them from retracting. This will minimize one of the great problems that repeatedly makes secondary nerve repair more difficult—the gap between the two ends. In a fresh nerve injury, even though there has been no loss of nerve substance, this gap is present because the nerve ends retract due to the elasticity in the mesoneurium. In order to restore continuity, it is often necessary initially to place gentle traction on both ends of the nerve to bring them together. If the nerve is to be repaired primary, the next step is to prepare the fresh ends. The dissecting microscope has the distinct advantage of allowing the surgeon to study these to see if all damaged and devitalized tissue has been removed prior to the repair. If the pneumatic tourniquet is being used and there is no colour contrast, the extent of damage is often difficult to evaluate. Many surgeons find it helpful to use a diluted mixture of methylene blue in order to improve this contrast along the cut margin. Very little is needed, and this can be applied to the cut nerve end with a sterile toothpick. This helps to outline the epineurium and the nerve bundles more clearly.

Before suturing, each interface must be prepared so that it will be flat and approximate to the other without causing distortion, twisting or protrusion of any of the funiculi. For some of the larger nerves it is worth while to hold the nerve in a fixed position while cutting it so that the interface will be absolutely perpendicular to the long axis of the nerve. One way to do this is to wrap some Surgicel around the cut end of the nerve and cover it with a small, thin sheet of plastic. The Surgicel gives added stability to the nerve end and its bundles inside while the plastic further immobilizes the ends. It can be tightened around the nerve by applying a straight clamp along the base of the plastic. A razor blade or dermatome knife helps to make a good, clean transverse cut. The freshly prepared interface should then be studied with the dissecting microscope to be certain that it is satisfactory for approximation to the other end. Once the other has been prepared, the repair can be undertaken.

As the suturing is begun, it is important to try to re-establish the original relationships of the nerve ends. There are at least four ways in which this proper alignment can be restored and rotational error minimized. One aid is to study the epineurial blood vessels on either side of the division and line them up. Another is to match up the mirror-like images of the nerve bundles in the cut ends. Sometimes there is a small groove or other difference in the contour on either side which will help. Finally, the mesoneurium normally extends down from the underside of a nerve to its underlying bed. Even if the mesoneurium is not intact at the site of nerve injury, remnants of it can be identified and used as a guide in correcting rotational error.

Magnification is advantageous both in the repair of large and small nerves. In the larger mixed nerve, it aids in preventing rotational errors and in securing the proper alignment of motor and sensory funiculi. In the smaller nerves, it is important because it aids in a more accurate closing of the epineurium. It seems that if the epineurium of a digital nerve is closed accurately so that there is no gap through which a funiculus can protrude, the chance of a painful neuroma at the site of nerve repair is markedly reduced. This is especially important in the fingers, where the amount of subcutaneous tissue is limited and is less than adequate for padding if the nerve is not properly repaired.

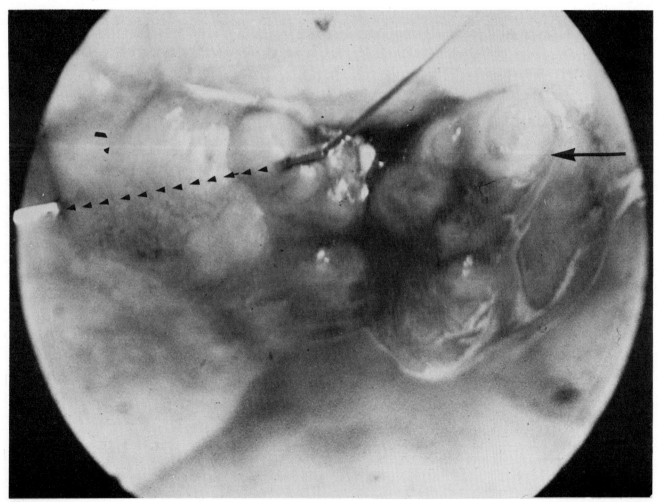

Figure 14.1
One arm of a double armed monofilament black nylon 'skewer' suture is shown (broken line) being placed into the perineural tissue to help stabilize the large fasciculus adjacent to it. The other end of the suture will be inserted into the perineural tissue of the opposing interface at the corresponding location (see arrow).

In the past most authors have suggested placing 'guide sutures' through the epineurium to aid in aligning it properly. It is further suggested that a straight needle be inserted through the nerve trunk several inches proximal and distal to the nerve juncture to take the tension off the juncture during the repair. As a substitute for this we have been inserting funicular guide sutures of nylon as the initial step before approximating nerve ends. These are placed through the epineurium about one centimetre back from the cut end and run horizontally down the nerve through the perineurium to the cut surface of the nerve (Fig. 14.1). A corresponding site is selected on the other cut end of the nerve and the guide suture passed down along the perineurium and out through the epineurium in just the reverse order in which it was inserted. If two to four sutures of this type (7–0 nylon) are accurately inserted they can be used in the realigning and also will serve well as traction or 'stay-sutures' to pull the ends together for the repair.

Epineurial guide sutures are placed accurately, one on each side of the nerve, but slightly more on its anterior surface, about 120 degrees apart. For the palm or the finger in an adult, a 7–0 nylon suture might be needed to overcome the tension. If 7–0 silk is used for the repair, it should be lubricated by running it through adjacent fat. Attention should again be directed to lining up the 'mirror-like patterns' of the funiculi so that any discrepancy in rotation is corrected as these sutures are placed into the epineurial sheath (Fig. 14.2). Once they are tied, light tension is placed upon them by clamping the ends of the suture with small mosquito clamps or a small lead weight. This will aid in

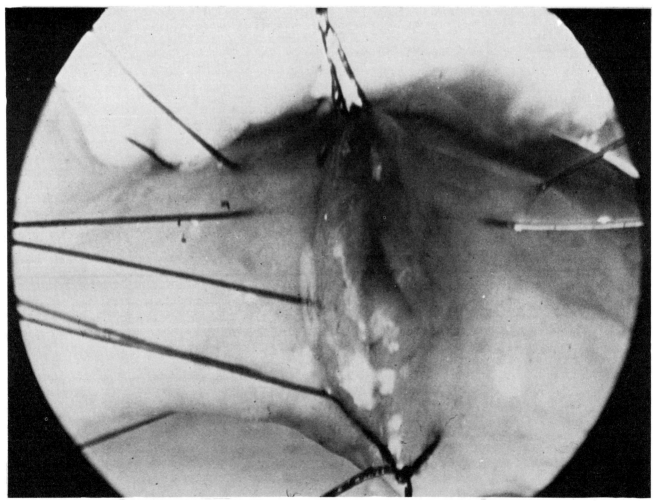

Figure 14.2
After several 'skewer' sutures are in place, only a few simple additional sutures are needed to approximate the adjacent connective tissue (epineurium or perineurium) and complete the repair. Note the fasciculi remain in better alignment with this technique at the site of repair even though there are only a few epineural sutures in place.

spreading out the epineurium at the site of repair and lining it up so that suturing is easier. The anterior repair should be performed first with a 7–0 or 8–0 microsurgical suture and then the posterior repair. This is carried out as follows: after the suturing is completed anteriorly, one of the epineurial guide sutures is drawn beneath the nerve and the other over the top so the nerve repair on the posterior side can be completed. If these epineurial guide sutures have been placed 120 degrees apart, the posterior margins of the sheath will remain slightly separated, a technical factor which greatly aids in identifying and more accurately closing the sheath on this side.

At the completing of the suturing, it is important to inspect the line of juncture to be sure that there are no defects in the epineurium through which funiculi can protrude. If the suture line is rolled between the fingers in the manner that a cigarette is rolled, this will further facilitate the lining up of the funiculi. The funiculi guide sutures on each side of the repair can be threaded onto a large cutting needle and passed out through the skin (Fig. 14.3). They can be tied to one another after the wound is closed. These funiculi guide sutures are removed at 7 days if the oedema and early stages of healing have fixed the funiculi to one another at the site of nerve juncture (Fig. 14.4).

Splinting of the extremity should hold it in such a position so that there will be no tension on the nerve ends during the 3 to 6 weeks of healing.

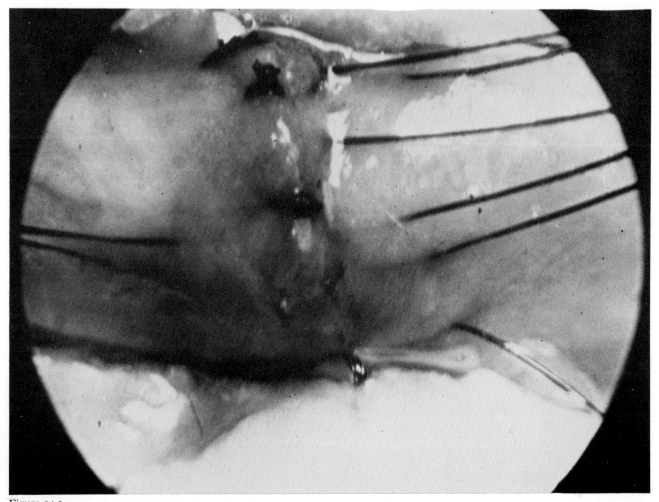

Figure 14.3
Completed closure. The perineural 'skewer' sutures maintain the internal configuration of the nerve and prevent fasciculi from kinking or falling out of alingment with one another. Since the epineural sutures are sufficiently strong to prevent the juncture from separating, the nylon sutures, which are brought out through the skin and tied loosely, can be removed at 7 days.

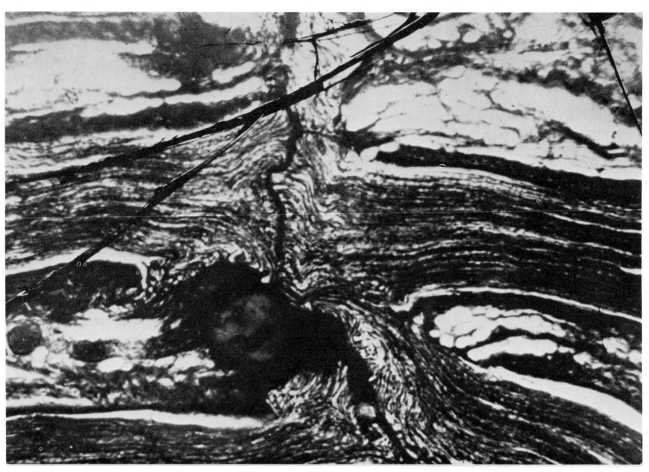

Figure 14.4
A photomicrograph demonstrates that a far better contact between fasciculi can be achieved with perifascicular 'skewer' sutures. Clinical experience supports these findings.

15. NERVE GRAFTING

Donal Brooks

Nerve grafting now occupies an established place in the surgery of peripheral nerves. Much of the credit for achieving this status must go to the pioneers in this work, namely Seddon, Young, Saunders and St Clair Strange in Great Britain, and Bunnell, Ballance, Duel and Woodall in the United States of America. It took the stimulus of the Second World War to provide the necessary impetus to perfect the technique of nerve grafting. Severe gunshot wounds of the extremities faced the surgeon with the problem of restoring continuity in nerves where large gaps had resulted from gross destruction of tissue and in which it was not possible to effect a repair by direct suture.

At that time the record of nerve grafting was indeed gloomy. In retrospect it is easy to see why the earlier attempt at nerve grafting were unsuccessful. There was a failure to appreciate the principles that apply to all peripheral nerve surgery; often nerves were repaired many months or even years after the original injury, when irreversible changes had taken place in paralysed muscles which precluded any hope of motor recovery. Resection of the neuroma was frequently inadequate, thereby hindering axonal regeneration. A single strand of a cutaneous nerve was used to bridge a gap in a main nerve trunk, thus seriously limiting the number of regenerating axons. Finally the use of homografts which had proved so successful in animal experiments were found to be quite useless in man, because of the reaction of immunity which they produced.

INDICATIONS FOR NERVE GRAFTING

Most surgeons accept that end to end suture still remains the method of choice in the repair of divided nerves. However, the work of Millesi in Vienna suggests that it may be necessary to reconsider this point of view. In general terms, therefore, nerve grafting is required when nerve suture is either impossible or undesirable.

LARGE GAPS

Whereas it may be technically possible to close extensive gaps by mobilising a nerve on either side of the lesion and acutely flexing one or more joints, the fact is that during postoperative stretching a traction lesion is inflicted on the nerve with subsequent intraneural fibrosis and little if any recovery. There is a biological rather than an anatomical limiting factor. As a practical guide it can be said that a nerve graft should be employed if the gap after mobilization cannot be closed by flexion of the main joint to a right angle, as for example the elbow, in lesions of the median and ulnar nerves, and the knee in the case of the sciatic nerve.

PARTIAL LESIONS

Lacerations in front of the wrist joint not uncommonly result in a partial loss of the median nerve, with sparing of motor or sensory function. At subsequent exploration a well-developed lateral neuroma in relation to intact nerve fibres is seen. In such circumstances after incision of the epineurium it is possible to separate damaged from intact nerve fibres. After resection of the neuroma the gap can be neatly bridged by means of an inlay graft.

EXCEPTIONAL CIRCUMSTANCES

In many hand injuries with concomitant nerve and tendon damage the optimum position of joint flexion for tendon repair rarely coincides with that suitable for nerve suture. Nerve grafting provides a means of overcoming this difficulty. Similarly when there is marked joint stiffness it may not be possible to close a gap after mobilization of the nerve, and here again grafting provides the only means of restoring continuity of the nerve.

FASCICULAR GRAFTING

In recent years Millesi has developed a technique of fascicular nerve grafting as an alternative to direct suture. It is his contention that failure after nerve suture can often be attributed to excessive tension at the suture line. Subsequent separation of the stumps occurs with the development of a haematoma, thereby causing a barrier to axonal regeneration. Nerve grafting enables restoration of fascicular continuity without tension. His results so far are very encouraging.

PRINCIPLES OF NERVE GRAFTING

Cutaneous nerves are usually employed for grafting material. The common donor in the upper limb is the medial cutaneous nerve of the forearm taken from the upper arm; in the lower limb, the sural nerve. Other nerves such as the radial nerve in the forearm, and the saphenous nerve in the lower limb can be used, but the area of sensory loss is often disagreeable to the patient.

Such cutaneous nerves have a cross-sectional diameter of 2–3 mm and yield an average of 22–30 cm of graft before breaking up into their terminal branches.

It sometimes happens that two main nerves are extensively damaged at the same time; in these circumstances part of the less important nerve may be used to graft its fellow.

Free nerve grafts are revascularised across their suture lines and also from the bed in which they lie. In the early stages this latter means of survival is probably the more important of the two. The metabolic requirements of a free graft in which the axons and myelin are still present were thought to be higher than one in which these materials had been previously removed by phagocytosis. It has been argued, therefore, that predegenerate grafting material should be used in preference to normal nerve. Nevertheless it has been shown that the results after the use of pre-degenerate grafts are not significantly better.

At one time it was considered that whereas axons might traverse the proximal suture line into the graft their progress at the far end was barred by fibrous invasion of the distal suture line from the surrounding tissues. It was suggested by Davis and Cleveland that the time taken for the axons to traverse the graft should be calculated and at the time that they were reckoned to have reached the distal suture line a resection and suture at this level should be undertaken. Furthermore, it was recommended that in order to prevent a fibrous invasion of the suture line, it should be wrapped with tantalum foil. However, the histological work of Abercrombie and others have shown that Schwann cell activity is greatest in the distal stump so that the distal junction is in fact the better of the two. Furthermore, surrounding the suture line with any material such as tantalum foil defeats its own object, not only by provoking a fibrous reaction but also by isolating part of the graft from its vascular bed. It is possible that the alleged fibrous invasion of the distal suture line was due in fact to a partial separation. It is known that considerable shortening of a free graft occurs after transplantation.

In summary, therefore, the general principles that apply to all peripheral nerve surgery with regard to adequacy of resection of stumps and time that has elapsed since the injury, must be observed. The cross-sectional area of the graft or grafts must be equal to that of the nerve to be repaired; the graft should be 12–15 per cent longer than the gap to be filled in order to allow for shrinkage; and finally the bed for the graft must be free from scar tissue to facilitate revascularization.

OPERATIVE TECHNIQUE

TYPES OF GRAFT

1. digital—free graft.
2. inlay—free graft.
3. cable—free graft.
4. interfascicular—free graft.
5. main trunk—free or pedicle graft.

Digital Grafts. Lacerations in the palm of the hand in addition to damaging flexor tendons may divide the digital nerves. In these instances our preference is for repair of the tendons before considering nerve repair, unless direct suture is possible. In those cases in which there are large gaps in the nerves, but where tendon repair is possible, nerve repair should be delayed until tendon function has been restored.

At a second operation the damaged nerve ends are excised and the gaps bridged by a strand of the medial cutaneous nerve of the forearm taken from the upper arm. It may be possible to suture the graft into position with 7–0 virgin silk, but it is often easier to 'glue' the ends together with plasma clot derived from a mixture of Thrombin and Fibrinogen. Care must be taken to localize the clots to the suture lines as otherwise revascularization of the graft is impeded. Unfortunately the bed for such a free graft is not ideal. Furthermore in addition to damage to the digital nerve, Seddon has shown that the digital vessels are often involved at the same time, giving rise to ischaemic changes in the distal segment of the nerve.

Postoperatively the hand is immobilized in a 'boxing glove' dressing and finger movements are discouraged until 3 weeks have elapsed from the time of nerve repair.

Inlay Grafts. Partial lesions of the median nerve at the level of the wrist give rise to a well developed lateral neuroma. At operation it is often possible to separate the damaged from the intact nerve fibres. Extra magnification such as that obtained by an operating microscope can be very helpful on these occasions. After resection of the lateral neuroma the gap is bridged by a strand or strands of cutaneous nerve and secured by plasma clot or very fine sutures.

Cable Graft. A cable graft composed of several strands of a cutaneous nerve is used to bridge a gap in a main nerve trunk such as the median nerve in the forearm, or the upper trunk of the brachial plexus, when direct suture is impracticable. It should be emphasised that the cross-sectional diameter of the cable graft must, of course, be equal to that of the main trunk. In nerves of large diameter, therefore, a considerable length of grafting material may be required. It has not been felt justifiable to use more than one donor nerve in any given case. In order to reduce the gap as much as possible it may be necessary to mobilize the nerve with optimum flexion of the neighbouring joint in addition to carrying out cable grafting. Fixation of the grafts can be carried out either by fine nerve sutures or by the use of plasma clot.

In certain circumstances it may be found necessary to carry out a cable graft when plasma clot fixation is not available. Provided the nerve grafting material is not immersed in saline prior to use, it will be found possible to approximate the strands of cutaneous nerve to the main trunk. They will adhere by the normal clotting process that takes place in the wound. In such circumstances a few fine sutures may be inserted.

Main Trunk—Free Graft. Clearly this type of nerve grafting is necessarily restricted, as it implies simultaneous damage to two main nerves. It also implies that direct suture of either nerve is impracticable. Gunshot wounds and industrial accidents are often associated with gross destruction of nerves and muscles in the forearm. In these instances restoration of continuity by direct suture is not possible. The nerve subserving the less important function can therefore, be used to graft its fellow. In the upper limb, for example, the ulnar nerve is used to graft the median nerve, to restore sensibility in the most important part of the hand. Similarly in the lower limb the lateral popliteal nerve can be used to repair the medial popliteal to restore protective sensibility in the sole of the foot and some action in the calf muscle. In such instances a free graft is taken from either the proximal or distal stump of the donor nerve, whichever is most convenient, and sutured into position using epineural sutures of some non-absorbable material such as fine white silk or human hair. As has been emphasized earlier, a free graft derives much of its blood supply from the bed in which it lies and clinical experience shows that the length of the graft is hardly relevant; the diameter is all important. The survival of a graft whose diameter is greater than the average median nerve, may experience difficulties in revascularization. It is for this reason that the bed in which the grafts lie is so important. It is often possible to by-pass a scarred area of muscle by rerouting the graft subcutaneously.

Main Trunk—Pedicle Graft. In severe Volkmann's anoxia of the forearm muscles the median and ulnar nerves are frequently destroyed over a considerable distance. Nerve suture is impossible. A main trunk graft taken from the ulnar nerve could not survive as a free graft because of the extensive scarring of the forearm muscles. It is in these very severe lesions in which conditions for free nerve grafting could hardly be worse that the pedicle nerve graft advocated by St Clair Strange has proved so helpful. The principles of pedicle nerve grafting are similar to those that apply to grafting of the skin. At the first stage the proximal neuromata of both nerves are resected and the ends sutured together. The extent of the gap to be closed in the median nerve is calculated. The ulnar nerve is then exposed in the upper arm, and allowing for some shrinkage, the level at which the nerve must be divided is calculated.

If possible the epineural vessels are dissected free from the nerve and the nerve is crushed at the appropriate level. It is convenient for future identification to tie a thick black silk suture around the nerve at the level at which it has been crushed.

The second stage is carried out not less than 6 weeks later. The ulnar nerve is again exposed in the upper arm, divided completely, and mobilized to the point at which the two nerves have been previously united. The nerve graft is then passed subcutaneously in the forearm to the distal stump of the median nerve exposed at the wrist joint. After resection of the stumps, the nerves are repaired in the usual way.

Homogenous Grafts. Homografts have been briefly referred to earlier and summarily dismissed. Within the last few years the subject has been revived again by Campbell, Marmor and others. The work has been largely carried out in animals the results being encouraging. However, time and time again it has been shown that it is not possible to transfer the results of animal experimentation to human beings. Furthermore before this method of nerve repair can be accepted it must be shown that the quality and regularity of recovery is better than that seen after conventional nerve suture and nerve grafting. At present no such evidence has been forthcoming.

16. TREATMENT OF NERVE LESIONS BY FASCICULAR FREE NERVE GRAFTS

H. Millesi

INTRODUCTION

Many papers have been published on nerve regeneration. The behaviour of the cells of Schwann, the outgrowing of the axons and other specific problems have been extensively studied. On the other hand only slight attention has been paid to the role of the connective tissue during healing of the nerve lesion. Both ends of a divided nerve are reconnected by connective tissue which is scar tissue. Krücke named this scar in accordance with its irregular structure 'Kontinuitätfibrom' (1955, 1967). The axons must pass through this scar during the process of nerve regeneration It is also supposed that the axons having passed the sutured part of the nerve will grow with a relatively constant speed distally in order to arrive at the end organ or structure.

It is accepted that the rate of the axonic growth varies between 1 and 4 millimeters each day.

EXPERIMENTS

In order to gain a better knowledge about the process of healing, specifically of the role of the connective tissue, a number of experiments have been carried out, which have been previously described (Millesi, Meissl, Berger) from other research centres. Therefore we will refer here only to the results of these experiments. The experimental animals were in one series cats and in the rest rabbits. The sciatic nerves of both hind limbs were divided and then reconnected using different techniques. The end result of the reconstruction was evaluated in the light of clinical and morphological characteristics. In each case both nerves from the same animal were compared in order to exclude individual factors. The results were also related within one group of animals, which had been operated upon under identical experimental conditions.

A total of 146 experimental animals were used and 252 nerve reconstructions during a relatively short time were made. The results of the experiments are thus summarized:

1. The extent of proliferation of the connective tissue is related to the tension at the site of the suture. The greater the tension, the greater the scarring at the site of the sutures (Figs. 16.1, 16.2).

2. There is also a direct relationship between the length of the scar between both nerve ends (Fig. 16.3) and the tension.

3. The proliferation of the connective tissue comes from the epineural, perineural and endoneural tissue. The epineural tissue produces the major part of the proliferative connective tissue. This connective tissue starts growing at the site of the suture, passing obstacles such as sutures on their outer side displacing them inwards. On the third day the site of suture is already encapsulated by a fibrinous membrane. After 8 days one can demonstrate a membrane of collagenous connective tissue.

4. The budding of the regenerating axons already takes place by the third postoperative day. If there is no obstacle the axons do not show any aberrant tendencies. Even when the axons have reached the distal stump of the divided nerve it can by no means be taken for granted that they will reach the actual end organs. Especially after tight nerve suture we could notice 5–9 weeks postoperatively, degenerative signs in the reconnected distal nerve-end in the regenerated axons. One can assume that there is shrinkage through scarring at the site of the nerve suture (Fig. 16.4).

5. Autogenous nerve grafts do survive transplantation. After 3–4 weeks the cells of Schwann are collected into bundles of Büngner and thus offer good conditions for the axons to pass.

6. Experiments with tension on nerves in situ have shown that for coaptation of the ends of the sharply divided sciatic nerve of the rabbit one needs a tension force of 5 to 6 grams. If the nerve ends are strained even more such as when it is necessary (Fig. 16.5) to overcome a gap caused by a tissue defect, the force necessary to connect the nerve ends at first rises slowly, but when about 4 per cent of the free length of the nerve stumps is reached the curve will rise very steeply. Thus return of the function was not at all good in that group of rabbits where there had been an excision of more than 4 per cent of the free nerve length, compared to the group where less suture tension was needed. Regenerating axons passed more easily through two lines of suture and 5 millimeters long nerve grafts than through a single line of sutures tied under tension. The best clinical and morphological results were obtained, after a single cut through

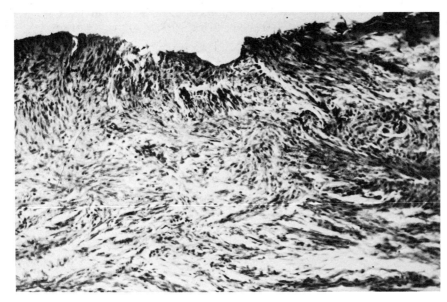

Figure 16.1
Rabbit no. 302. The sciatic nerve seen 2 weeks postoperatively on the one hand (a) after suturing with tension and on the other after a nerve grafting (b).
Htx van Gieson. Magnification 1:31,5.

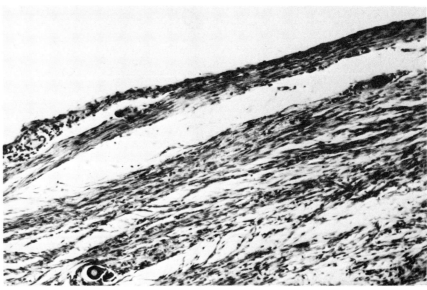

Figure 16.1A clearly shows a more extensive connective tissue proliferation, as compared to 16.1B.

the sciatic nerve, when a nerve graft, equal in length to the gap between the retracted sciatic nerve ends was sutured into place without any tension exactly filling the gap and gave nerve regeneration with a minimum of connective tissue proliferation. The regeneration so obtained was almost equal to isomorphic axon growth.

7. The connective tissue originating from the epineurium, growing along the nerve distally, surrounded the epineural sutures pushing the sutures into the nerve tissue in a centroneural direction and thus there was loss of part of the neural diameter required for the regeneration. Therefore the number of sutures should be limited to a minimum and the finest, i.e. thinnest possible suture material used. Practically, this is possible only in coaptation without tension.

8. With epineural sutures under tension we very often noticed a sliding of the sutures distally to the free end of the proximal perineurium. This was made possible by the greater elasticity of the epineurium (Sunderland, 1968). Loose epineural suturing is dangerous because of the risk of an inner separation of the fascicles although there is a preservation of the epineural continuity. This may cause a greater amount of connective tissue between the nerve ends. If, on the other hand, one ties the epineural sutures too tightly, a displacement of the single fascicles of the transsected nerve will be seen and so one will have such

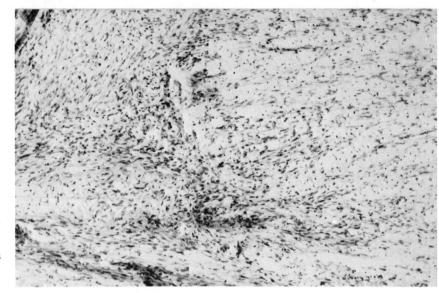

Figure 16.2A
Rabbit no. 302. The same sciatic nerve as in Fig. 18.1.
Htx van Gieson. Magnification 1:31.5.

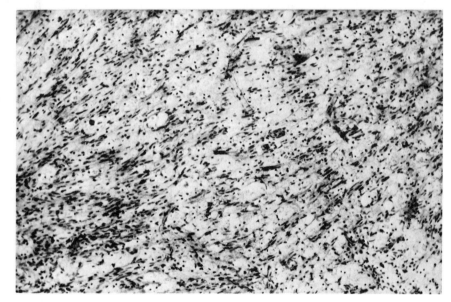

After suturing with tension there is at the site of the anastomosis a centrally located separation, which is not seen (Fig. 16.2B) when the sutures have been tied without tension.

pictures as were published by Edshage (1964). The phenomenon of the displacement is accentuated by the propulsion of the endoneural tissue from the perineural cylinder. We do not think it is possible to get a really smooth, cut surface with a better technique. By the protrusion of the endoneural tissue there will always be irregularities in the cut surface. The above mentioned greater elasticity of the epineural tissue makes the fascicular coaptation even more difficult. One must therefore seriously pose the question of whether there is any justification in suturing the epineural sheath and if it wouldn't be better to resect it proximally and distally to the suture line, in order to minimize the bulk of proliferating connective tissue.

9. Heiss and Faul (1965) published good results after reconnection of experimentally divided nerves in the rabbit with the help of artificial glueing materials (Butylcyanoacrylat). Our experiments (Berger, Millesi and Gangelberger, 1967) showed that regeneration which started and went on well after five weeks showed degeneration in the already regenerated axons due to extensive connective tissue proliferation around the cement deposits. The same thing happened even if we very cautiously avoided contamination between cement and nerve tissue.

10. We have also tried experimentally to wrap the sutures with collagen and silastic sheaths (Campbell and Luzio, 1964, Ducker and Hayes, 1967, 1968; Lehmann and

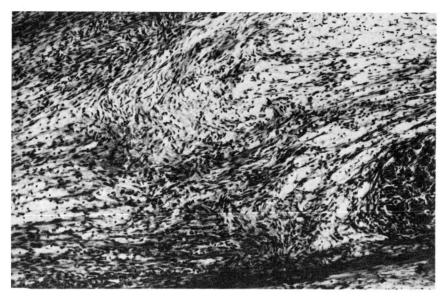

Figure 16.3
Rabbit no. 5. The suture line of the sciatic nerve 30 days after suturing with tension. Htx van Gieson. Magnification 1:31.5.
    Between the nerve ends the diastasis is clearly filled by connective tissue.

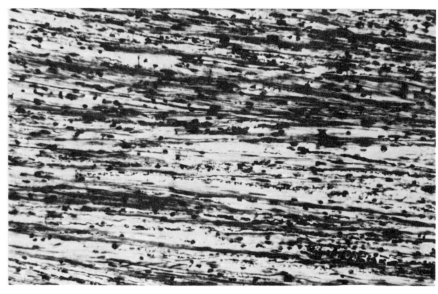

Figure 16.4
Rabbit no. 53. The distal stump of the sciatic nerve. Bodian. Magnification 1:78.7. Thirty-two days after a nerve suturing with tension, regenerated axons are clearly demonstrable in the distal stump, and some of these show signs of recent degeneration.

Hayes, 1967; Kline and Hayes, 1964; Freeman, 1965. The results were far behind the expected ones. Between the nerve and the above mentioned sheath there was an extensive connective tissue proliferation. Thus the epineural connective tissue proliferation cannot be stopped by means of wrapping. A suture line without tension will very soon be overgrown, at first on the third day by a fibrinous membrane, then by collagenous connective tissue on the eighth day. There is under these conditions no risk either of aberration of the axons or of ingrowth by surrounding connective tissue. Only when the connection is made under tension to close a gap does connective tissue ingrowth take place. There is only a limited value in 'the wrapping up

method' and only so if the sutures are placed without tension.

CLINICAL EVIDENCE

All our experimental results indicate that one of the most important factors to be avoided in the process of healing of nerve structures and in neural tissue regeneration is tension on the suture line. This very important role is generally accepted and stressed by all authors. It was, however, believed that one could arrange suture without tension by means of mobilization of the nerve and flexion of the adjacent joints in order to overcome a defect in the nerve.

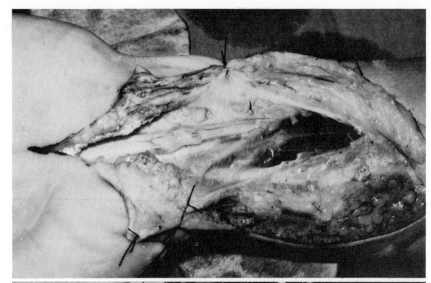

Figure 16.5
A, Case with a complete loss of function in the median nerve area after a glass cut: At the operation 4 weeks after the injury both ends of the nerve are held together by scar tissue.
B, The epineural tissue was then excised just leaving a dorsal strip in order to prevent a separation of the nerve stumps. Both nerve stumps were then dissected into single bundles of fascicles.
C, The fascicular arrangement on the cut surface of the nerve ends was then outlined on paper, enabling the identification of corresponding fascicles. The scar tissue between the nerve stumps was then excised, and the corresponding bundles of fascicles were joined by free nerve grafts.

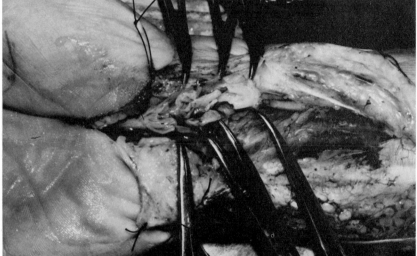

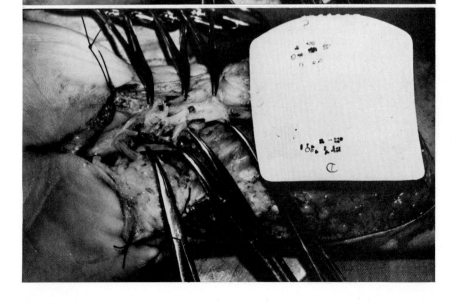

The critical length thus possible to overcome, varies in the literature between 5 and 16·5 centimetres (Nafziger, 1921; Forester-Brown, 1921; Babcock, 1927; Grantham *et al.*, 1947; Seddon, 1948; Zachary, 1954; Highet and Sanders, 1943; Sunderland, 1968; Nulsen, 1968). Fixation of the adjacent joint favours the process of healing and will thus prevent a rupture or a separation. Sooner or later the joint fixation has to be removed and even if cautiously and gradually extended over a long time there will be a continuous tension exerted on the sutures which is then followed by connective tissue proliferation at the line of sutures. With scars in the skin we can observe this phenomenon very clearly and there is no reason to assume that connective tissue scarring in the skin should differ from that in the nerve. On the contrary, our experimental work has demonstrated the direct connection between connective tissue proliferation and tension exerted on the suture line.

There would be no reason for fear, if one could assume that the axons, which have just passed the line of suture, would not be harmed through the process of scarring. On the contrary, our experiments have shown, that regenerated axons will be harmed in this way and show signs of degeneration. Observations in experiments with animals should not be uncritically applied to human beings. Thus we have made histological studies on ten human nerve sutures, which were made under moderate tension and where regeneration did not take place. In seven of these ten cases one could demonstrate in both directions an even greater disseminated degeneration of the nerve fibres beyond the suture line. In all ten cases there were suture granulomata more or less blocking the regeneration of the nerve and in all ten cases there was extensive connective tissue proliferation. In two cases no axon regeneration had reached the distal stump. Five times, however, a single regenerating axon had passed through the suture line, but in each case it was insufficient to evoke clinical recovery.

In three patients the axons had grown into the distal stump and showed a high percentage of degenerative alterations which was still in a progressive phase although 8–12 months had passed since the nerve suture. These observations confirmed the experimental findings. Therefore one must take into account that even after a so-called suture without tension, with the joint fixed in flexion, regeneration will not take place, since tension not only

can cause rupture or displacement at the suture line but also by secondary scarring may exert a harmful effect on the outgrowing axons, which have already grown into the distal stump of the cut nerve.

The relationship between the length of the defect and the end result of the nerve suture is published in many papers. So Nicholson and Seddon (1957) and Sakellarides (1962) put the upper limit of a defect at 2·5 centimetres beyond which one can expect the results to deteriorate.

SURGICAL TECHNIQUE

These experimental results and also experience with conventional suture techniques gave us the stimulus to alter our surgical technique: (Fig. 16.6).

The injured epineurium of the proximal and distal stump is first resected, and then the single fascicles were isolated from the injured part of the nerve. This preparation has to go up to the point of dissection beyond which we find uninjured tissue or secondary contracted scar tissue. The dissection of the single fascicles takes place step by step in injured, unscarred tissue. Larger fascicles at the cut surface of the nerve are isolated and smaller adjacent fascicles are left together in groups or bundles. The fascicles are thus transected step by step at different levels along the nerve. The intraneural vessels are ligated with 10-0 nylon or microcoagulated. We proceed in the same way at the distal stump. The operating microscope greatly facilitates this preparation.

Then a sketch is made of the cut surface of both the proximal and the distal ends and after this mapping we have a guide for the identification of corresponding fascicles and bundles of fascicles. In short defects this is not very difficult. If the defects are longer we will see an even greater difference in the arrangement of the fascicles on the two cut surfaces. If one joins the fascicles of the corresponding quadrants there is a good chance that some of the fibres of the proximal quadrant are guided into the right peripheral pathway. Here the topographic facts found by the experiments of Sunderland come in although he has made different deductions.

We think, in opposition to Sunderland's views, that one has to cut through into absolutely unharmed tissue since

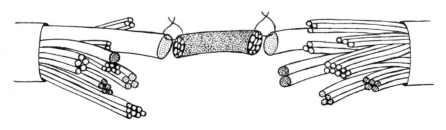

Figure 16.6
Schematic drawing of an interfascicular nerve grafting. After excision of the epineurium and the dissection of the nerve ends into single, corresponding bundles of fascicles, they are then joined with the help of nerve grafts. In this operation seven single nerve grafts were used. The cut surfaces are exact fit for each other and are anchored with the help of single sutures of nylon 10-0.

every connective tissue scar left in the cut surface will be an obstacle to regeneration. If in doubt, resect. The operating microscope will help to determine whether all injured or scarred tissue has been resected.

If there is no defect or a defect of less than 1·5–2·0 centimetres one can with mobilization of tissue get an attachment without tension. The corresponding fascicles are one by one joined and adapted by two perineural sutures per fascicles or group of fascicles (nylon 10-0).

In larger defects a nerve suture will be made only when it is possible to suture without tension. For example by transposing the ulnar nerve at the elbow or by shortening a limb by means of bone resection in a case of pseudarthrosis. In all other cases the bridging of the defect should be made by a nerve transplant (Fig. 16.7). One can obtain whole nerves only when there has been, or if there will be, an amputation of a limb. In free transplants of thick nerves there is a risk of central necrosis developing before reconnection of central circulation.

In other cases nerve grafting is not feasible due to loss of function at the donor site. In a case where two nerves in a limb are severed there is justification for reconstruction of one of the nerves taking tissue from the other. Of course one has to abandon the reconstruction of this donor nerve. Successful use of homografts are frequently reported in papers (Weiss, 1943; Weiss and Taylor, 1943; Lyons and Woodhall, 1949; Nulsen et al., 1959; Marmor, 1963; 1964, 1967; Böhler, 1961, 1962; Campbell et al., 1961; Iselin, 1967). The neurotization of preserved homotransplants takes place in the following way. A regenerating neuroma will grow through the transplant (Schröder and Seiffert, 1970). These authors have coined the concept of neuromatous neurotization. Seiffert et al. (1968) report the distance thus passed at 4–5 centimetres. As in autotransplants

not only the connective tissue cells but also the Schwann cells survive this mode of transplanting, which facilitates neurotization. With preserved homotransplants one puts in a skeleton of connective tissue without living cells. Bielschofsky and Unger (1917) recommend thin cutaneous nerves as donors. Various methods have been worked out in order to join several thin cutaneous nerves to make a single cable transplant of the right calibre for the size of the nerve to be repaired. This was done either with suturing or with cementing of cutaneous nerves with plasma (Bunnell and Boyes, 1939; Young and Medawar, 1942; Tarlow, 1945). With the help of the cable transplants there was reported regeneration i.e. return of meaningful function in 50 per cent of the cases (Sanders, 1942; Seddon, 1954; Brooks, 1955). We have also used such cable grafts. Since 1964 our technique of transplanting a nerve has been changed in the following way:

We don't try any more to join the single cutaneous nerve strands to a thick cable. The single strands are used to join corresponding fascicles or bundles of fascicles, which were isolated as outlined above. The transplants are exactly the length of the tissue defect or preferably just a bit longer.

Our first choice of a donor nerve is the small nerves of both lower extremities, secondly the medial cutaneous nerve of the forearm. Both nerves can easily be found and obtained through small transverse incisions. The sural nerve corresponds in thickness to the cut surface of either one bigger, or three to four smaller fascicles of a mixed nerve of the upper extremity (Fig. 16.8). The free ends of the transplants are apposed directly to the cut surface of the corresponding fascicle or bundles of fascicles and an exact fit obtained using the operating microscope.

As no tension exists the grafts will stick very well to the cut ends of the corresponding fascicles. This position is

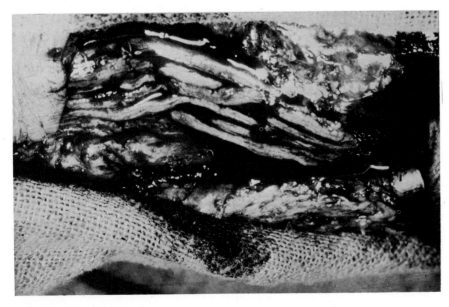

Figure 16.7
Interfascicular nerve grafting procedure is here bridging a 12 cm long defect of the median nerve.

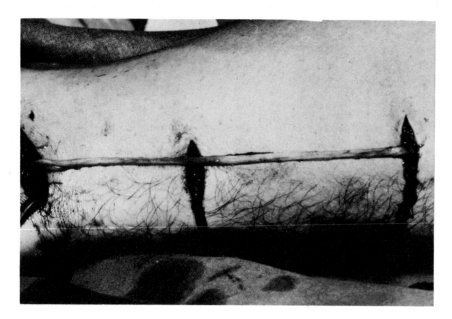

Figure 16.8
The sural nerve is located with a small incision behind the fibular malleolus and then followed proximally. It is visualized through several skin incisions and finally excised.

secured with one or at the most two fine stitches of 10-0 nylon at both free ends of the transplant. The perineurium of the fascicle is joined to the epineurium of the grafts. As the fascicles or bundles of fascicles were divided at various levels along the nerve a serrated apposition at both ends of the transplant will add to the security of junction.

The single transplants have a relatively large surface area in contact with the corresponding recipient bed which offers a very good chance for survival.

As there is no tension whatsoever on the suture line the whole operation is performed with the least possible surgical trauma. Digital nerves correspond in calibre to a piece of the sural nerve so that here a fascicular dissection is not necessary and the graft can be interposed between the free ends of the divided digital nerve. In more proximal parts of the peripheral nerves, for example, at the level of the brachial plexus, the cut surface is composed of many small fascicles. A fascicular dissection as mentioned above is not possible and we have to rely on epineural suturing.

RESULTS

Since 1964, 194 peripheral nerves in 160 patients have been operated upon in a manner mentioned above with a total sum of 202 nerve reconstructions (Tables 1, 2). The results of 70 reconstruction operations on nerves in the upper extremity, including the hand, are shown in the table in the appendix. The cases are all old enough to make a final evaluation of the results possible. Only cases were included where reconstruction was made not later than 2 years after the injury and where there were no innervational anomalies present. With one exception, they are all secondary reconstructions.

In a great majority of the cases, the optimal time was missed and it was too late for an early secondary reconstruction. On many patients there have been one or two previous operations without success. With two exceptions the defect in continuity was more than 3 centimetres in length. The length of the various defects can be studied in the tables. In the follow-up all were free from neuromas and paraesthesias (Tables 3, 4 and 5).

The motor function was classified using Highet's scheme. The return of sensitivity was classified with the two-point discrimination test, where alas contrary to Moberg a paper clip was not used but an instrument with two sharp points as had been originally promoted by Weber. In many cases

TABLE 1

Plexus brachialis	21	22
N. fac.	1	1
N. ophth.	1	1
N. acc	1	1
N. axill.	5	5
N. musculocut.	1	1
N. rad.	16	16
N. med.	42*	45
N. uln.	42*	43
N. dig.	28	49
N. femoral	1	1
N. fibularis	11	12
N. tib.	1	1
N. isch.	3	4
	160	202

* In fourteen cases both the ulnar and median nerve in the same arm had been injured.

on follow-up there was a fairly acceptable two-point discrimination. A grouping of so-called 'ideal' cases, following Moberg's proposal, showed a better return of two-point discrimination ability than would have been expected having used Önne's scheme (Fig. 16.9).

These ideal cases had had complete median or ulnar lesions where defects of up to 11 centimetres were bridged by nerve transplants. The local wound state, the patient's age and the time elapsed since the denervation (Table 9) were here favourable factors.

TABLE 2

	Number of cases	Too short to evaluate	Sufficient	Axon growth	Axon growth after resection of the distal suture line	Successful Yes	Successful No	No axon growth
Plexus	21	4	17	12	2		1	2
N. fac.	1		1	1				
N. ophth.	1	1						
N. acc.	1		1	1				
N. axill.	5		5	3				2
N. musc.	1		1	1				
N. rad.	16	4	12	11				1
N. med.	43	10	33	29	2	1	1	
N. uln	42	10	32	26	3	1	1	2
N. dig.	46	3	43	40		2	1	
N. fém.	1		1	1				
N. fib.	11	2	9	8		1		
N. tib.	1	1						
N. isch.	3		3	1		1		1
	193	35	158	134	7	5	4	8

134 + 7 = 141
141 + 5 = 146 ; 4 + 8 = 12

TABLE 3

Return of motor function
N. median 16
N. cubital 18
N. radial 6

	M 0	M 1	M 2	M 2+	M 3	M 4–5
N. median	—	—	1	—	6	9
N. cubital	—	—	1	3	6	8
N. radial	—	—	—	—	1	5
	—	—	2	3	13	22
Length of the grafts						
− 5 cm	—	—	1	1	7	13
−10 cm	—	—	—	—	4	7
−15 cm	—	—	—	1	1	2
−20 cm	—	—	1	1	1	—
Patient's age						
−19a	—	—	—	1	3	10
−39a	—	—	—	1	4	7
−59a	—	—	2	1	4	3
60−a	—	—	—	—	2	2

TABLE 4

Return of sensibility
N. median 16
N. cubital 18

	0	Dysesthesia	Protective function	2PD > 10 mm	2PD < 10 mm
N. med.	—	—	9	1	6
N. cubit.	—	1	10	1	6
Length of the grafts					
− 5 cm	—	1	10	1	7
−10 cm	—	—	5	1	2
−15 cm	—	—	2	—	2
−20 cm	—	—	2	—	1
Patient's age					
−19a	—	—	2	2	8
−39a	—	—	6	—	4
−59a	—	1	7	—	—
60−a	—	—	4	—	—

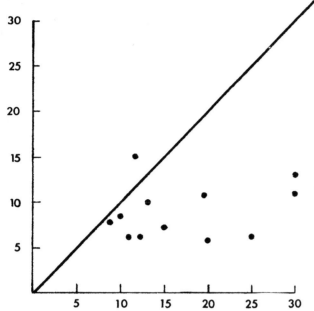

Figure 16.9
Return of two-point discrimination in twelve 'ideal' cases. Nerve repair was carried out by free grafting according to the interfascicular technique. Listed according to the suggestion of Moberg.

TABLE 5

	Number of patients	Number of nerve grafts
Plexus brachial	21	22
N. fac.	1	1
N. ophth.	1	1
N. acc.	1	1
N. axill.	5	5
N. musculocut.	1	1
N. radial	16	16
N. median	42*	45
N. ulnar	42*	43
N. digital	28	49
N. femoral	1	1
N. peroneus comm.	11	12
N. tibial	1	1
N. sciat.	3	4
	160	202

* In fourteen cases both the ulnar and median nerve in the same arm had been injured.

Our above mentioned results are not unique. In several centres the techniques of interfascicular nerve transplantation is also in use and good results have been reported (Buck-Gramcko, 1970; Palazzi, 1970; Samii and Willebrand, 1970). Also Verdan and Narakas (1968) reported surprisingly good results.

SUMMARY

The avoidance of any tension at the site of the sutures seems to be the most important factor influencing the regeneration of divided peripheral nerves. Tension must be avoided not only during the immediate healing phase but also later as scar processes can be deleterious to already regenerated axons. The regenerating axons pass through two lines of sutures and a graft, without tension, much easier than through a single suture line under tension. The author's own procedure in reconstructing divided peripheral nerves is described in detail as well as the late postoperative results.

BIBLIOGRAPHY

ABERCROMBIE, M. & JOHNSON, M. L. (1942). The outwandering of cells in tissue cultures of nerves undergoing Wallerain degeneration. *Journal of Experimental Biology*, **19**, 266.

ADAMS, W. E. (1943). The blood supply to nerves. II. The effects of exclusion of its regional sources of supply on the sciatic nerve in rabbit. *Journal of Anatomy*, **77**, 253.

ALMQUIST, E. E. & OLOFSSON, E. (1972). Bilan électrique et clinique des sutures nerveuses en fonction de l'âge. Monographie du G.E.M. (Groupe d'Etude de la Main), *Lésions traumatiques des Nerfs périphériques*. Paris: Expansion Scientifique Française.

ASCHAN, W. & MOBERG, E. (1962). The ninhydrin finger printing test used to map out partial lesions to hand nerves. *Acta chirurgica scandinavica*, **123**, 365.

AULICK, L. A. (1967). The galvanic-tetanus ratio test: an evaluation of the tetanus standard. *Physical Therapy*, **47**, 933.

BABCOCK, W. (1927), A standard technique for operations on peripheral nerves with special reference to the closure of large gaps. *Surgery, Gynaecology and Obstetrics*, **45**, 364.

BALLANCE, CH. & DUEL, A. M. (1932). Operative treatment of facial palsy by the introduction of nerve grafts into the Fallopian canal and by other intratemporal methods. *Archives of Otolaryngology*, **15**, 1.

BASSET, A., WACKENHEIM, A. & CROSSHANS, E. (1969). La neurographie lipiodolée du nerf cubital. Lèpre. Tumers. Acropathie ulcéromutilante. *Annales de Radiologie*, **12**, 565.

BATEMAN, J. E. (1962). *Trauma to nerves in limbs*. London: Saunders.

BAUWENS, P. (1942). Heat and electricity in the treatment of nerve lesions. *British Journal of Physical Medicine and Industrial Hygiene*, **5**, 48 and 96.

BENJAMIN, R. & THOMPSON, R. (1959). Differential effect of cortical lesion in infant and adult cats on roughness discrimination. *Experimental Neurology* **1**, 305.

BENTLY, F. H. & HILL, M. (1936). Experimental Surgery. Nerve grafting. *British Journal of Surgery*, **24**, 368.

BERGER, A., MEISSL, G. & SAMII, M. (1970). Experimentelle Erfahrungen mit Kollagenfolien über nahtlose Nervenanastomosen. *Acta neurochirurgica, Vienna*, **23**, 141.

BERGER, A., MILLESI, H. & GANGLBERGER, J. (1967). Experimentelle Untersuchungen zur Nervennaht mit Klebstoffen. I. *Internationale Kongress für Klebstoffe*, Wien, September 1967.

BIELSCHOWSKY, M. & UNGER, E. (1916–18). Ueberbruckung grosser Nervenlucken. Beitrage zue Kenntnis der Degeneration und Regeneration peripherer Nerven. *Journal of Physiology and Neurology*, **22**, 267.

BISCHOFF, A. (1969). The ultrastructure of the peripheral nervous system. In *Ultrastructure of the Peripheral Nervous System and Sense organs*. Stuttgart: Thieme.

BISHOP, G. H. (1960). Relation of nerve fiber size to modality of sensation. *Advances in Biology of Skin*. Vol. 1. *Cutaneous Innervation*. New York: Pergamon Press.

BJÖRKESTEN, G. (1947). Suture of war injuries to peripheral nerves. *Acta chirurgica scandinavica*, Suppl. 119.

BLUNT, M. J. (1959). The vascular anatomy of the median nerve in the forearm and hand. *Journal of Anatomy*, **93**, 15.

BÖHLER, J. (1962). Nervennaht und homioplastische Nerventransplantation mit Milliporeumscheidung. *Referat gehalten am 28.4.1962 bei der Tagung der Deutche Gesellschaft für Chirurgie in München*.

BÖHLER, J. (1963). Weitere Erfahrungen mit der Mikrofilterumscheidung von Nervennähten und von homioplastischen Nerventransplantaten. *Langenbecks Archiv für klinische Chirurgie*, **304**, 944.

BÖHLER, J. (1966). Nerventransplantation und Tubulisation von Nervennahten und Nerventransplantation. In *XV Congrès de la Société Internationale de Chirurgie Orthopaédique et de Trauamatologie*, Paris.

BOSWICK, J. A., Jr., Schneewind, J. & STROMBERG, W., Jr. (1965). Evaluation of peripheral nerve repairs below elbow. *Archives of Surgery*, **90**, 50.

BOURREL, P., BOURGES, M. & GIRAUDEAU, P. (1969). Neurolyse du neft tibial posterieur au canal tarsien dans le traitement des maux perforants plantaires lepreux. *Annales de Chirurgie plastique*, **14**, 341.

BOWDEN, R. E. M. & NAPIER, J. R. (1961). The assessment of hand function after peripheral nerve injuries. *Journal of Bone and Joint Surgery*, **43 B**, 481.

BRAIN, R. (1962). *Diseases of the Central Nervous System*. London: Oxford University Press.

BRAND, P. W. (1966). Tendon transfers in the forearm. In *Hand Surgery* (edited by J. E. Flynn). Baltimore: Williams & Wilkins.

BRANES, G. K., SHAFFER, D. V., WAKIM, K. G., SAYRE, G. P. & KRUSEN, F. H. (1954). Quantitative observations on skeletal muscle undergoing denervation atrophy. *Archives of Physical Medicine*, **35**, 689.

BROOKS, D. (1955). The place of nerve grafting in orthopaedic surgery. *Journal of Bone and Joint Surgery*, **37 A**, 299.

BUCHWALD, J. S. (1947). Proprioceptive reflexes and posture. *American Journal of Physical Medicine*, **46**, 104.

BUNNELL, S. (1927). Surgery of the nerves of the hand. *Surgery, Gynaecology and Obstetrics*, **44**, 145.

BUNNELL, S. & BOYES, J. H. (1939). Nerve grafts. *American Journal of Surgery*, **45**, 64.

CAJAL, S. R. (1909). *Histologie du système nerveux*. Paris: Maloine.

CAMPBELL, J. B. (1966). Discussion in *Xe Congrés de la Société internationale de chirurigie orthopèdique et de traumatologie*. Paris.

CAMPBELL, J. B., BASSETT, C. A. L., HUSBY, J., THULIN, C. A. & FERINGA, E. R. (1961). Microfilter sheaths in peripheral nerve surgery: a laboratory report and preliminary clinical study. *Journal of Trauma*, **1**, 139.

CAMPBELL, J. B. & LUZIO, J. (1964). Symposium: facial nerve rehabilitation. Facial nerve repair: new surgical techniques. *Transactions of the American Academy of Ophthalmology and Oto-laryngology*, **68**, 1086.

CARAYON, A., FAYE, I., COURBIL, L. J. & RESILLOT, A. (1965). Indications de la neurographie pour névrite hansenienne. *Bulletin de la Société médicale d'Afrique noir de langue française*, **10**, 121–124.

CARPENDALE, M. (1966). The localization of ulnar nerve compression in the hand and arm—an improved method of electroneuromyography. *Archives of Physical Medicine*, **47**, 325.

CAVE, L., FUSTEC, R. & BASSET, A. (1965). Radiologie de la le'pre. *Annales de Radiologie*, **6**, 61–76.

CAVE, L., FUSTEC, R., BASSET, A., FAYE, I. & COURSON, B. (1965). Cent neurographies cubitales chez des Hanseniens. *Bulletin de la Société médicale d'Afrique noir de langue française*, **10**, 101–120.

CHASE, R. A. (1960). Management of nerve injuries in the upper extremity. *Surgical Clinics of North America*, **40**, 287.

CLIPPINGER, F. W., GOLDNER, J. L. & ROBERTS, J. M. (1962). Use of the electromyogram in evaluation upper extremity peripheral nerve lesion. *Journal of Bone and Joint Surgery*, **44 A**, 1047.

COWAN, J. (1940). The treatment of nerve injuries. *British Journal of Physical Medicine*, **3**, 118.

DANIELS, L., WILLIAMS, M. & WORTHINGHAM, C. (1964). *Evaluation de la fonction musculaire. Le 'testing'; techniques de l'examen manuel*. Paris: Maloine.

DAVIS, L. & CLEVELAND, D. A. (1934). Experimental studies in nerve transplants. *Annals of Surgery*, **99**, 271.

DE LORME, T. L. (1945). Restoration of muscle power with heavy resistance exercise. *Journal of Bone and Joint Surgery*, **27**, 654.

DE LORME, T. L. & WATKINS, A. L. (1948). Technique of progressive resistance exercise. *Archives of Physical Medicine*, **29**, 263.

DE LORME, T. L. & WATKINS, A. L. (1951). *Progressive Resistance Exercise*. New York: Appleton-Century-Crofts.

DEYERLE, W. W. M. & TUCKER, F. (1960). Tendon transplants in the wrist following nerve injury. *Southern Medical Journal*, **53**, 1562.

DENNY-BROWN, D. (1966). Electromyography and other electrical aids to diagnosis. In *Hand Surgery* (edited by J. E. Flynn). Baltimore: Williams & Wilkins.

DOBBELSTEIN, H. & STRUPPLER, A. (1963). Die Nervenleitungsgeschwindigkeit als diagnostiches Kriterium dei peripheren neurologischen Storungen. *Fortschritte der Neurology und Psychiatrie und ihrer Grenzgebiete*, **31**, 616.

DOUPE, J., BARNES, R. & KERR, A. S. (1943). Studies in denervation. The effect of electrical stimulation on the circulation and recovery of denervated muscle. *Journal of Neurology and Psychiatry*, **6**, 136.

DOWNIE, A. W. (1969). Studies in nerve conduction. In *Disorders of voluntary muscles* (edited by J. Walton). London: Churchill.

DOWNIE, A. W. & SCOTT, T. R. (1964). Radial nerve conduction studies. *Neurology*, **14**, 839.

DUCHENNE, G. B. A. (1949). *Physiology of Motion*. (translated by E. M. Kaplan). Philadelphia: Lippincott.

DUCKER, T. B. & HAYES, G. J. (1967). A comparative study of the technique of nerve repair. *Surgical Forum*, **28**, 443.

DUCKER, T. B. & HAYES, G. J. (1968). Peripheral nerve injuries: a comparative study of the anatomical and functional results following primary nerve repair of chimpanzees. *Military Medicine*, **133**, 298.

DYER, L. (1964). Rehabilitation following peripheral nerve injuries. *Physiotherapy*, **50**, 61.

EDSHAGE, S. (1964). Peripheral nerve suture. A technique for improved intraneural topography. *Acta chirurgica scandinavica*, Suppl. 331.

EDSHAGE, S. (1968). Peripheral nerve injuries—diagnosis and treatment. *New England Journal of Medicine*, **278**, 1431.

ENTIN, M. A. (1964). Restoration of function of paralysed hand. *Surgical Clinics of North America*, **44**, 1049.

FENG, T. P. & LIU, Y. M. (1949). The connective tissue sheath of nerve as an effective diffusion barrier. *Journal of Cellular and Comparative Physiology*, **34**, 1.

FERNÁNDEZ-MORÁN, H. (1950). Sheath and axon structures in the internode portion of vertebrate myelinated nerve fibres. An electron microscopic study of rat and frog sciatic nerves. *Experimental Cell Research*, **1**, 309.

FLYNN, A. F. (1966). Peripheral nerve injuries in the hand. In *Hand Surgery* (edited by J. E. Flynn). Baltimore: Williams & Wilkins.

FOERSTER, O. (1929). *Symptomatologie der Schussverletzungen der peripheren Nerven*. Berlin: Springer.

FORREST, W. J. (1967). Motor innervation of human thenar and hypothenar muscles. *Canadian Journal of Surgery*, **10**, 196.

FORRESTER-BROWN, M. (1921). The possibilities of suture after extensive nerve injury. *Journal of Orthopaedic Surgery*, **19**, 277.

FREEMAN, B. S. (1965). Adhesive neural anastomosis. *Plastic and Reconstructive Surgery*, **35**, 1967.

GAMBLE, H. J. & GOLDBY, S. (1961). Mast cells in peripheral nerve truncs. *Nature* (Lond.), **189**, 766.

GAMSTORP, I. & SHELBURNE, S. A. (1965). Peripheral sensory conduction in ulnar and median nerves of normal infants, children and adolescents. *Acta paediatrica scandinavica*, **54**, 309.

GARDINER, M. D. (1963). *The Principles of Exercise Therapy*. London: Bell.

GASSEL, M. M. (1964). Sources of error in motor nerve conduction studies. *Neurology*, **14**, 825.

GAUJOUX, E., LAVIELLE, J., PICHERAL, J. F. & VACHERAR, S. (1969). La neurographie à contraste lourde des grow troncs nerveux du mêmbre supérieur. *Journal de Radiologie et d'Electrologie*, **6, 553**.

GEREN, B. C. (1954). The formation from the Schwann cell surface of myelin in the peripheral nerves of chick embryos. *Experimental Cell Research*, **7**, 558.

GRANTHAM, E. G., POLLARD, C., Jr. & BRABSON, J. A. (1948). Peripheral nerve surgery: repair of nerve defects. *Annals of Surgery*, **127**, 696.

GRAY, H. G. (1959). *Anatomy of the Human Body*, p. 1017. Philadelphia: Lea & Febiger.

GUTH, L. (1956). Regeneration in the mammalian peripheral nervous system. *Physiological Reviews*, **36**, 441.

GUTMANN, E. & GUTTMANN, L. (1942). Effect of electrotherapy on denervated muscles in rabbits. *Lancet*, **i**, 169.

GUTMANN, E. & GUTTMANN, L. (1944). The effect of galvanic exercise on denervated and reinnervated muscles in rabbit. *Journal of Neurology, Neurosurgery and Psychiatry*, **7**, 7.

HEISS, W. H. & FAUL, P. (1965). Nervennaht mit Klebstoff. *Langenbecks Archiv klinishe Chirurgie*, **313**, 710.

HIGHET, W. B. & SANDERS, F. K. (1943). Effects of stretching nerves after suture. *British Journal of Surgery*, **30**, 355.

HURSH, J. B. (1939). Conduction velocity and diameter of nerve fibers. *American Journal of Physiology*, **127**, 131.

ISELIN, M. & ISELIN, F. (1967). *Traité de chirurgie de la main*. Paris: Flammarion.

JACKSON, S. (1945). The role of galvanism in the treatment of denervated voluntary muscle in man. *Brain*, **68**, 300.

JACKSON & SEDDON, H. J. (1945). Influence of galvanic stimulation on muscle atrophy resulting from denervation. *British Medical Journal*, **ii**, 485.

JOHNSON, E. W. & OLSEN, J. K. (1960). Clinical value of motor nerve conduction velocity determination. *Journal of the American Medical Association*, **72**.

JUUL-JENSEN, P. & MAYER, R. F. (1966). Threshold stimulation for nerve conduction studies in man. *Archives of Neurology* (Chicago), **15**, 410.

KABAT, H. (1961). Proprioceptive facilitation in therapeutic exercise. In *Therapeutic Exercise*. Baltimore: Waverly Press.

KEMBLE, F. & PEIRIS, O. A. (1967). General Observations on sensory conduction in the normal adult median nerve. *Electromyography*, **7**, 127.

KEY, E. H. & RETZIUS, G. (1876). *Studien in der Anatomie des Nervensystems und Bindegewebes*. Stockholm: Samson & Wallin.

KLINE, G. & HAYES, G. J. (1964). The use of resorbable wrapper for peripheral repair nerve. *Journal of Neurosurgery*, **21**, 968.

KNOTT, M. & VOSS, D. E. (1960). *Proprioceptive Neuromuscular Facilitation. Patterns and Techniques*. New York: Hoeber-Harper Books.

KOSMAN, A. J., OSBORNE, S. L. & IVY, A. C. (1947). The influence of duration and frequency of treatment in electrical stimulation of paralysed muscle. *Archives of Physical Medicine*, **105**, 571.

KRÜCKE, W. (1955). Erkrankungen des peripheren Nervensystems. In *Handbuch der spezielle pathologiste Anatomie und Histologie*, Berlin: Springer.

KRÜCKE, W. (1967). Aur Morphologie der Erkrankungsformen peripherer Nervenfasern. *Chirurgica plastica et reconstructiva*, **31**, 1.

LAFRATTA, C. W. (1964). An appraisal of electrodiagnostic testing. *Southern Medical Journal*, **57**, 649.

LANGE, M. (1953). Die Behandlung der irreparablen peripheren Nervenen letzungen. *Wiederherstellungschizurgie und Traumatologie* **1**, 240.

LAING, P. G. (1960). The timing of definite nerve repair. *Surgical Clinics of North America*, **40**, 303.

LANDSMEER, J. M. F. (1962). Power grip and precision handling. *Annals of Rheumatic Diseases*, **21**, 164.

LARSEN, R. O. & POSCH, J. L. (1958). Nerve injuries in the upper extremity. *Archives of Surgery*, **77**, 469.

LEFFERT, R. D. & FRAENKEL, V. H. (1963). The value of determination of conductive velocity of peripheral nerves in orthopaedic surgery. *Bulletin of the Hospital for Joint Diseases*, **25**, 32.

LEHMANN, H. J. (1953). The epineurium as a diffusion barrier. *Nature* (London), **172**, 1045.

LEHMANN, R. A. & HAYES, G. J. (1967). Degeneration in peripheral nerve. *Brain*, **90**, 285.

LIU, C. T. & LEWEY, F. H. (1947). The effects of surging currents of low frequency in man on atrophy of denervated muscles. *Journal of Nervous and Mental Diseases*, **105**, 571.

LIU, C. T., SANDS, O. E. & SOWEY, E. M. (1948). Tensile strength of human nerves. *Archives of Neurology and Psychiatry*, **59**, 433.

LOVETT, R. W. (1917). *The Treatment of Infantile Paralysis*. Philadelphia: Blackstone.

LYONS, W. R. & WOODHALL, B. (1949). *Atlas of Peripheral Nerve Injuries*. Philadelphia: Saunders.

MACCABRUNT, F. (1911). Der Degenerationsprocess der Nerven bei der homoplastischen und heteroplastischen Propfung. *Folio neuro-biologica*, **5**, 1911.

McEWAN, L. E. (1962). Median and ulnar nerve injuries. *Australian and New Zealand Journal of Surgery*, **32**, 89.

MANNERFELT, L. (1966). Studies on the hand in ulnar nerve paralysis. *Acta orthopaedic scandinavica*, Suppl. 87.

MARMOR, L. (1963). Regeneration of peripheral nerve defects by irradiated homografts. *Lancet*, **i**, 1191.

MARMOR, L. (1964). Regeneration of peripheral nerves by irradiated homografts. *Journal of Bone and Joint Surgery*, **46 A**, 383.

MARMOR, L. (1967). *Peripheral nerve regeneration using nerve grafts*. Springfield, Illinois: Thomas.

MAYER, R. F. (1963). Nerve conduction studies in man. *Neurology*, **13**, 1021.

MELVIN, J. G. L., HARRIS, D. & JOHNSON, E. W. (1966). Sensory and motor conduction velocities in the ulnar and median nerves. *Archives of Physical Medicine and Rehabilitation*, **47**, 511.

MEIROWSKY, A. M. (1965). *Neurological Surgery of Trauma*. Washington: U.S. Army Medical Service.

MENNELL, J. (1942). Massage, movements and exercises in the treatment of nerve suture and repair. *British Journal of Physical Medicine*, **5**, 40.

MICHON, J. (1972). La suture nerveuse en 1971. Monographie du G.E.M. (Group d'Etude de la Main), *Lesions traumatiques des Nerfs peripheriques*. Paris: Expansion Scientifique Française.

MILLESI, H., GANGLBERGER, J. & BERGER, A. (1967). Erfshrungen mit der Mikrochirurgie peripherer Nerven. *Chirurgie plastica et reconstructiva*, **3**, 47.

MILLESI, H. (1969). Wiederherstellung durchtrennter peripherer Nerven und Nerventransplantation. *Münchener medizinische Wochenschrift*, **111**, 2669.

MILLESI, H. (1972). Traitement des lésions nerveuses par greffes fasciculaires. Monographie du G.E.M. (Group d'Etude de la Main), *Lésions traumatiques des Nerfs périphériques*. Paris: Expansion Scientifique Francaise.

MILLESI, H., BERGER, A., GANGLBERGER, J. & GESTRING, F. G. *Ergebnisse der interfascicularen Nerventransplantation*.

MILLESI, H., BERGER, A. & MEISSL, G. (1970). Entwicklungstendensen in der operativen Wiederherstellung durchtrennter peripherer Nerven. *Bolesti i Ozljede Sake Medicinska*. Zagreb: Naklada.

MITCHELL, S. W., MOREHOUSE, S. R. & KEE, W. W. (1864). *Gunshot Wounds and other Injuries of Nerves*, Philadelphia.

MOBERG, E. (1958). Objective methods of determining the functional value of sensibility of the hand. *Journal of Bone and Joint Surgery*, **40 B**, 454.

MOBERG, E. (1960). Examination of sensory loss by the ninhydrin printing test on Volkmann's contracture. *Bulletin of the Hospital for Joint Diseases*, **21**, 296.

MOBERG, E. (1962). Criticism and study of methods for examining sensibility of the hand. *Neurology*, **12**, 8.

MOBERG, E. (1964). Aspects of sensation in reconstructuve surgery of the upper extremity. *Journal of Bone and Joint Surgery*, **46 A**, 817.

MOBERG, E. (1964). Handchirurgie. *Klinische Chirurgie für die Praxis*. Stuttgart: Thieme.

MOBERG, E. (1966). Methods of examining sensibility of the hand. In *Hand Surgery* (edited by J. E. Flynn). Baltimore: Williams & Wilkins.

MOBERG, E. (1968). Nerve repair in hand surgery. *Surgical Clinics of North America*, **48**, 985.

MOBERG, E. (1972). Akute Handchirurgie. Stuttgart: Thieme.

MURPHY, F. (1963). Peripheral nerve injuries. In *Campbell's Operative Orthopaedics*, chap. 23. St. Louis: Mosby.

NAFFZIGER, H. C. (1921). Methods to secure end-to-end suture of peripheral nerves. *Surgery, Gynaecology and Obstetrics*, **32**, 193.

NAPIER, J. R. (1956). The prehensile movements of the human hand. *Journal of Bone and Joint Surgery*, **38 B**, 902.

NARAKAS, A. & VERDAN, C. L. (1969). Les greffes nerveuses. *Zeitschrift für Unfallmedizin und Berufskrankheiten*, **137**.

NEWMAN, M. R., BERRIS, J. M. & BOHN, S. S. (1940). Management of facial paralysis by physical measures. *Archives of Physical Therapy*, **21**, 270.

NICHOLSON, O. R. & SEDDON, H. J. (1957). Nerve repair in civil practice. Results of treatment of median and ulnar nerve lesions. *British Medical Journal*, **ii**, 1065.

NORDENBOOS, W. (1959). *Pain*. Amsterdam: Elsevier.

NULSEN, F. E. (1966). The management of peripheral nerve injuries producing hand dysfunction. In *Hand Surgery* (edited by J. E. Flynn). Baltimore: Williams & Wilkins.

NULSEN, F. E., LEWIEY, F. H. & VAN WAGEB, W. (1959). *Peripheral Nerve Injuries* (edited by Spurlig & Woodhall). Washington: U.S. Government Printing Office.

OFFNER, F. (1946). Stimulation with minimum power. *Journal of Neurophysiology*, **9**, 238.

OMER, G. E. (1956). The early management of gunshot wounds of the extremities. *South Dakota Journal of Medicine and Pharmacy*, **9**, 340.

ÖNNE, L. (1962). Recovery of sensibility and sudomotor activity in the hand after nerve suture. *Acts Chirurgica Scandinavica* Suppl., 300.

ÖNNE, L. (1964). Sensibility of the hand. The mechanism of cutaneous sensibility. *Current Practice in Orthopaedic Surgery*, **2**.

POLLOCK, L. J. (1927). *Motor disturbances in peripheral never lesions*. The Medical Department of U.S. Army. Washington: Government Printing Office.

RANVIER, L. (1878). *Leçons sur l'histologie du système nerveux*. Paris: Sary.

ROBERTS, J. TH. (1948). The effect of occlusive arterial diseases of the extremities on the blood supply of nerves. *American Heart Journal*, **35**, 369.

ROBERTSON, J. D. (1955). The ultrastructure of adult vertebrate peripheral myelinated nerve fibres in relation to myelinogenesis. *Journal of Biophysical and Biochemical Cytology*, **271**.

SAKELLARIDES, H. (1962). A follow-up study of 173 peripheral nerve injuries in the upper extremity in civilians. *Journal of Bone and Joint Surgery*, **44 A**, 140.

SAMII, M. & WILLEBRAND, H. *Zur Indikation und mikrochirurgischen Technik autologen Nerventransplantaten*. In print.

SANDERS, F. K. (1942). The repair of large gaps in the peripheral nerves. *Brain*, **65**, 281.

SANDERS, F. K. & YOUNG, J. Z. (1942). The degeneration and reinnervation of grafted nerves. *Journal of Anatomy (London)*, **76**, 143.

SCHRAMM, D. A. (1967). Resistance exercise. In: *Therapeutic exercise*. Baltimore: Waverly Press.

SCHRÖDER, J. M. & SEIFFERT, K. E. (1970). Die Feinstruktur der neuromatosen Neurotisation von Nerventransplantaten. *Virchows Archiv für pathologische Anatomie und Physiologie und für kenische Medizin*, **5**, 219.

SEDDON, H. J. (1943). Three types of nerve injury. *Brain*, **66**, 237–228.

SEDDON, H. J. (1947). The use of autogenous grafts for the repair of large gaps in peripheral nerves. *British Journal of Surgery*, **35**, 151.

SEDDON, H. J. (1948). War injuries of peripheral nerves. *British Journal of Surgery*, Suppl. 2, 325.

SEDDON, H. J. (1954). *Peripheral nerve injuries*. London: Her Majesty's Stationery Office.

SEDDON, H. J. & HOLMES, W. (1944). Ischemic damage in the peripheral stump of a divided nerve. *British Journal of Surgery* **32**, 389.

SEIFFERT, K. E., SCHINDLER, P., THOMES, E., SCHRÖDER, M. & HUFSCHMIDT, F. (1968). Experimentelle Technik und Ergebnisse der homologen Nerventransplantation. *Lagenbeck's Archiv für klinische Chirurgie*, **322**, 598.

SEITELBERGER, F., SLUGA, E., MEISSL, G. & MILLESI, H. *Morphologische Untersuchungen an Nähten und Transplantationen nach Nervenläsionen*. In print.

SHAFFER, D. V., BRANES, G. K., WAKIM, K. G., SAYRE, G. P. & KRUSEN, F. H. (1954). The influence of electric stimulation on the course of denervation atrophy. *Archives of Physical Medicine*, **35**, 491.

SIMPSON, S. A. & YOUNG, J. Z. (1945). Regeneration of fibre diameter after cross-unions of visceral and somatic nerves. *Journal of Anatomy (London)*, **79**, 48.

SMITH, H. W. (1966). Factors influencing nerve repair. *Archives of Surgery*, **93**, 335.

SMITH, J. W. (1964). Microsurgery of peripheral nerves. *Plastic and Reconstuctive Surgery*, **33**, 317.

SPURLING, R. G., LYONS, W. R., WHITCOMB, B. B. & WOODHALL, B. (1945). The failures of whole fresh homogenous nerve grafts in man. *Journal of Neurosurgery*, **2**, 79.

SPURLING, R. B. & WOODHALL, B. (1946). Experience with early nerve surgery in peripheral nerve injuries. *Annals of Surgery*, **123**, 731.

STILLWELL, G. K. (1959). *Clinical electric stimulation*, p. 104. Baltimore: Waverley Press.

STOPFORD, J. S. B. (1918). The variation in distribution of cutaneous nerves of the hand and the digits. *Journal of Anatomy* (London), **53**, 14.

STRANGE, F. G. (1947). An operation for nerve pedicle grafting. *British Journal of Surgery*, **34**, 423.

SUNDERLAND, S. (1944). Voluntary movements and the deceptive action of muscles in peripheral nerve lesions. *Australian and New Zealand Journal of Surgery*, **3**, 160.

SUNDERLAND, S. (1945a). Blood supply of the nerves in the upper limb in man. *Archives of Neurology and Psychiatry* (Chicago), **53**, 91.

SUNDERLAND, S. (1945b). Blood supply of peripheral nerves: practical considerations. *Archives of Neurology and Psychiatry* (Chicago), **53**, 91.

SUNDERLAND, S. (1945c). The intraneural topography of the radial, medial and ulnar nerves. *Brain*, **68**, 243.

SUNDERLAND, S. (1947). Observations of the treatment of traumatic injuries of peripheral nerves. *British Journal of Surgery*, **35**, 36.

SUNDERLAND, S. (1952). Factors influencing the course of regeneration and the quality of recovery after nerve suture. *Brain*, **75**, 19.

SUNDERLAND, S. (1954). Funicular suture and funicular exclusion in the repair of severed nerves. *British Journal of Surgery*, **40**, 580.

SUNDERLAND, S. (1968). *Nerves and nerve injuries*. Edinburgh: Livingstone.

SUNDERLAND, S. & RAY, L. J. (1947). The selection and use of autografts for bridging gaps in injured nerves. *Brain*, **70**, 75.

SUNDERLAND, S. & BEDBROOK, G. M. (1949). The cross-sectional area of peripheral nerve trunks occupied by fibres representing individual muscular and cutaneous branches. *Brain*, **72**, 613.

TARLOW, I. M. (1950). *Plasma clot suture of peripheral and nerve roots*. Springfield, Illinois: Thomas.

TARLOW, I. M. & EPSTEIN, J. A. (1945). Nerve grafts: The importance of adequate blood supply. *Journal of Neurosurgery*, **2**, 49.

TACHDJIAN, M. O. & MINEAR, W. L. (1958). Sensory disturbances in the hands of children with cerebral palsy. *Journal of Bone and Joint Surgery*, **40 A**, 85.

TASAKI, L., ISHI, & ITO, H. (1943). On the relation between the conduction rate, the fibre-diamter and the internodal distance of the medullated nerve fibre. *Japanese Journal of Medical Science (III. Biophysico)*, **9**, 189.

TINEL, J. (1915). Le signe du Fourmillement dans le lésions des nerfs peripheriques. *Presse Médicale*, **47**, 388.

TINEL, J. (1917). *Nerve wounds: Symptomatology of peripheral nerve lesions caused by war wounds*. New York: Wood.

TUBIANA, R. (1969). Anatomic and physiologic bases for the surgical treatment of paralysis of the hand. *Journal of Bone and Joint Surgery*, **51 A**, 643.

TUBIANA, R. (1971). Traitement palliatif des paralysies des muscles du pouce. *Annales de Chirurgie*, **25**, 971.

VILANOVA, ST. (1948). La radiographia de los nerviose cubitales en los enformos de lepra. *International Journal of Leprosy*, **16**, 351.

VON FREY, M. & KIESOW, F. (1899). Ueber die Function der Tastkorperchen. *Zeitschrift für Psychologie*, **20**, 126.

VON PRINCE, K. (1966). Occupational therapy's interest in sensory function following peripheral nerve injury. *Medical Bulletin, U.S. Army, Europe*, **23**, 43.

Voss, D. E. (1967). Proprioceptive neuromuscular facilitation. *American Journal of Physical Medicine*, **46**, 838.

Wakim, K. G. & Krusen, F. H. (1955). The influence of electric stimulation on the work output and endurance of denervated muscle. *Archives of Physical Medicine*, **36**, 370.

Wakim, K. G. & Krusen, F. H. (1956). Studies on denervation atrophy and the effect of electrical stimulation on that atrophy. *Procedures of the Second International Congress of Physical Medicine in Copenhagen.*

Wakim, K. G. & Kruse, F. H. (1957). Comparison of effects of electric stimulation with effects of intermittent compression on the work output and endurance of denervated muscle. *Archives of Physical Medicine*, **38**, 21.

Weiss, P. (1943). Functional nerve regeneration through frozen-dried nerve grafts in cats and monkeys. *Proceedings of the Society for Experimental Biology (N.Y.)*, **52**, 326.

Weiss, P. & Taylor, A. C. (1943). Repair of peripheral nerves by grafts on frozen dried nerve. *Proceedings of the Society for Experimental Biology (N.Y.)*, **54**, 277.

White, W. L. (1960). Restoration of function and balance of the wrist and hand by tendon transfers. *Surgical Clinics of North America*, **40**, 427.

Whitecomb, B. B. (1959). Techniques of peripheral nerve repair. In *Peripheral Nerve Injuries* (edited by Spurling & Woodhall). Washington: U.S. Government Printing Office.

Woodhall, B. & Beebe, G. W. (1956). *Peripheral Nerve Regeneration*. Veterans Administration Medical Monograph. Washington: U.S. Government Printing Office.

Wynn-Parry, C. B. (1966). *Rehabilitation of the hand*. London: Butterworth.

Yeoman, P. M. (1964). Peripheral nerve injuries. *Physiotherapy*, **50**, 56.

Young, J. Z. & Medawar, P. B. (1940). Fibrin suture of the peripheral nerves: Measurement of the rate of regeneration. *Lancet*, **ii**, 126.

Zachary, R. B. (1954). Results of nerve suture. In *Peripheral Nerve Injuries* (edited by H. J. Seddon). London: H.M.S.O.

Zancolli, E. (1968). *Structural and dynamic cases of hand surgery*. Philadelphia: Lippincott.

AUTHOR INDEX

SUBJECT INDEX